C0-ANB-810

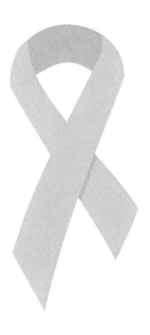

Breastless
But Still Breathing

A Breast Cancer
Survivor's Journey

By Anita DuJardin Hockers

with Kathleen Marie Marsh

ISBN: 0-9760796-2-3

Published by Otter Run Books LLC
16965 Nicolet Road, Townsend, WI 54175
www.otterrunbooks.com

Cover design by Joe Bergner
Cover photography by Drew Neerdaels

First Printing May 2006

Printed in the United States.

For Ray, my best friend

Acknowledgments

My thanks to my editor and friend, Kathleen Marsh, for her belief in me and my story; to John Maino for insisting that this book should not be hidden in a drawer, that it needed to be read; to Joe Bergner at Imaginasium for his time and expertise in designing the cover; to Drew Neerdaels at Launch Photography for his kindness and generosity; to Carol Nuthals at Steen Macek Paper for her friendship and donation; to Loralee Olson for her time in making my book "look" like a book; to the boys at FedEx Ground: Kevin, Luke, Adam, Andrew, Jamie and Marc, for making every day at work seem as "normal" as possible—here's to being bald together; to Dr. Mike, Dr. Colette and Dr. J, you saved my life with smiles and the best care possible; to my old and new friends, the ones who were at my side, you knew when I needed you.

My heartfelt thanks to Colette Siedl, my aunt, who is my "sister in cancer." Your constant presence and love was a gift of hope during some very dark days; to Jon and Matt, my brothers, you are loved; to Colleen DuJardin-Pricco, for loving me and listening to me. Thanks for letting me know that I indeed had a story to tell, like a handprint on my heart, I love you sister; to Sharon and Neil DuJardin, my Mom and Dad, for their love, unending smiles and encouragement; and to Alyce and Tony for continuing to think that their mom rocks.

**They put this poison into my body…
they injected drugs that would melt the floor into
my veins…but you grab at straws in the life and
death struggle with this monster…
you try anything…**

The magnitude of chemotherapy is overwhelming. I get sick every time I think of it. Just writing this makes me nauseous. They put this poison into my body. Do you understand? They injected drugs that would melt the floor into my veins to destroy the rapidly-growing cells that were trying to kill me. But what else were they killing? My hair…yes…but what else? Seriously, no one can understand, really understand, unless you've been there. I can still smell the drugs. I can still taste them.

"I cannot tell you how much this book meant to me. I HATE that it's a true story; but thank you, Anita, for writing it. I know it will help countless others cope with the beast called breast cancer. You are one HELL of a courageous woman!"

Patti Beske
Cancer-Caregiver

"An endearing story. Readers will connect with Anita on what it's like to live with a breast cancer diagnosis. Her honesty, humor, determination, and zest for life will surely touch your heart. Thank you for sharing your story and offering hope to those affected with breast cancer."

Kathy Miller
Ribbon of Hope Foundation

Contents

Introduction

We all know the statistics, or we should. This "cancer-thing" can happen to anyone. Breast cancer occurs mostly in women, but it can happen to men. It strikes among the young and the old. Women with a family history of breast cancer face an even greater risk of becoming a statistic.

With the alarming number of breast cancers being diagnosed, there are stories to tell. I sat down one day and decided that telling my story would be a tribute to my daughter, my family, my friends, and especially to those of you who will fall victim to this vicious disease.

When tough times pass, we tend to forget. Forgetting can be a good thing. Women forget how much it hurts to have a child, ex-spouses forget the pain of a nasty divorce, soldiers forget the trauma of war, and cancer survivors forget how long the months really are when we are fighting this disease.

But I do not want to forget. I am putting my foot down right here. Going to the edge of hell and stepping back was monumental. I want everyone, especially the one in seven who will be diagnosed with breast cancer, to know that there is an end, and they need to keep fighting!

After all, it's the fight that makes the difference. You will have hair again, although some of it could have stayed gone. You will regain your strength. You will have your own story to tell. Here is my story. I have not written anything like this before. My story is not unique, by any means, but it is worth reading because it is a story of survival. Surviving is what we do best, and we can make a difference.

Chapter 1

A Lump Doesn't Lie

*The true test of character is how we behave
when we don't know what to do.*
John W. Holt

While rolling over in bed one Friday morning in 2004, I felt a strange lump in my right breast. Still half-asleep, I explored it with my fingertips. It was BIG, about the size of a small egg. I was stunned. *It wasn't there a few days ago; I would definitely have felt it.*

Wide-awake now, I got out of bed as quietly as I could so I wouldn't wake up Ray. I went down to the kitchen to check my appointment calendar. It was August 13. *Friday the 13th. Doesn't that just figure?* I had a full day scheduled, and Ray wanted to leave for the cottage right after work. *No need to panic. It's probably just another cyst. I'll call Dr. Mike first thing Monday morning.*

I had always had issues with my boobs. Always. I was never proud of my breasts; in fact, I considered them an adversary that would do me in some day. When I would see models and actresses, or normal everyday women, showing off their surgically enhanced chests, I wasn't envious...*Wow, sure wish I had those!* I felt quite the opposite...*Man, what a pain in the ass.*

It's true. Ever since I had "developed," my breasts were a problem. I was a 38DD, and my breasts were fibro-cystic. They were always sore, and they always seemed to be in the way. Whether it was trying to find the right bra or trying to find a shirt that fit, they were trouble. Having dense and fibro-cystic breasts, I would do the self-exams and not know one bump or lump from another. But because I was so positive I would be a breast cancer patient some day, I was vigilant about doing the exams, booking annual physicals, and having mammograms.

What led me to the inevitable conclusion that I would have breast cancer? Genetics. My maternal grandmother Evelyn died at the age of 45 from breast cancer. My maternal great-grandmother Henrietta died at the age of 38 from breast cancer. My maternal great-great-grandmother Virginia, from what we are told, also died of breast cancer.

To trace the progression of my fight against this cruel disease back to its very beginning, I would have to say it started with a scare and a biopsy in December 2001. After a lumpectomy, that mass had turned out to be benign. Lucky me. I had a sneaky feeling that this was not going to be the story this time, but I decided not to even think about it during our weekend getaway to Door County.

It was a busy, fun-filled weekend, and I was successful at keeping my mind (and my fingers) off the lump. But when I awakened Monday morning, there was an unbidden feeling of dread in the pit of my stomach. I tentatively felt my breast, searching out the lump, praying it had disappeared as mysteriously as it had appeared. *Oh, God, it's still there; I have to call Dr. Mike.*

I fought back my rising panic, got Ray off to work, and went to work myself. I used a phone in the back office to call the clinic the minute they opened. Monday mornings are the busiest time of the week for medical offices, and it took a while to get through. When I finally got the receptionist and explained the situation, she scheduled an appointment for me that very afternoon.

Now let's just get this out of the way. I am practically the president of the "Dr. Mike Fan Club." He has always been the kindest doctor and one of the nicest men I have ever met. I am convinced it was no accident I found Dr. Mike. When I was in my mid-twenties, Ray and I were thinking about starting a family, and I needed to find an OB/GYN specialist. I grabbed a phone book, searched for a clinic near work, and happened upon his listing. I called; he was new to the area; he had openings. I immediately booked a physical. No referral, no background research, no initial consultation.

I will not say I am wrapped up in the belief that everything happens *for a reason*. I do not believe I got cancer *for a reason*. I cannot believe parents lose a child *for a reason*. I do believe that when we are born, we have a path, from A to B or maybe A to Z. We may take a wrong turn here or there, but inevitably, we get back on our path. I do not believe in luck, good or bad. I would hate to think that my life is based on chance. I do believe that a higher power determines our path and that this higher power knew I would need Dr. Mike.

When Ray and I had our daughter Alyce in 1990, Dr. Mike was not on call. I was so disappointed that he was not there to deliver my first baby. When it was time for Anthony to make his appearance in 1994, Dr. Mike made it to the hospital...bedhead and all...just in time to supervise the birth of our son.

Over the years, Dr. Mike has listened to my little complaints, always with a smile. He never seems to be in a hurry. When I call the office, he usually calls me back. Not one of his nurses; Dr. Mike himself. He finds time out of his busy day to ask about Ray, the kids, whatever else is on my mind. I don't know if he's like that with all of his patients, but I consider our relationship very special.

I have a tendency to grin and joke around when I'm nervous. I remember that I greeted Dr. Mike with my usual smile, even managing a couple of giggles. I recall the crinkling sound of the stiffly starched gown and the cold examining table when Dr. Mike asked me to lie down. He was very thorough, carefully inspecting the lump, manipulating it this way and that. I could tell by the way he looked at me that this wasn't going to end well, so I made an off-hand comment in a feeble attempt at humor. "I always knew these boobs were going to be the death of me."

Chapter 2
I Always Hated Tests

Difficult times have helped me to understand better than before, how infinitely rich and beautiful life is in every way, and that so many things that one goes worrying about are of no importance whatsoever...
Isak Dinesen

Dr. Mike knew how I felt about my breasts. He smiled at my joke and then looked me right in the eye, responding in an almost scolding tone. "None of that, Anita," he said. "You will not be dying anytime soon, not from your breasts or anything else." Then he called in his nurse and proceeded to aspirate the lump.

That's Step One: aspiration. From what I had been told during my earlier biopsy, an aspiration should produce fluid from the questionable area. If not, there could be a problem. I tried not to look when Dr. Mike numbed my breast and inserted a very large needle into the lump. He did not get any fluid. I could tell this was not the result he was hoping for. He ordered Step Two: a mammogram. Immediately.

"But, Dr. Mike," I protested as I sat up, "I just had a mammogram two months ago." It was standard procedure for me because of my family history: yearly physical and mammogram with a six-month check in between, just in case there were any changes. I had breezed through those exams for three years in a row with flying colors. *How can there be something wrong when it's only been two months? Oh, well, Dr. Mike knows best.* I obediently went to get another mammogram.

When the technician called me in, her demeanor was flat. Not cross, flat, like this was just another day on the job. I remember this because I really wanted her to say, *"This is going to be nothing."* I am sure she had done many mammograms on a moment's notice, and that most of them found nothing. Perhaps these technicians are trained to be emotionless, lest they give false hope in the event that the test does show something.

She started the familiar process. *Stand here. Get up on your tiptoes. Move a little more this way. Let me put your breast in this vice. Sorry if my hands are cold. Now stand still. I'm going to crank it a little at a time. The more compression, the better the picture. Let me know when you can't stand the pressure.* Crank. Crank. Crank. *Hold your breath. Count to five. Okay, breathe.* Sweet release. *Good work. All done. Get dressed and have a seat in the waiting room while the doctor checks the film.* Wait. Hurry up and wait. I sat. I waited. Then suddenly, I panicked. Alyce.

Before my appointment, I had picked up my daughter from a summer gym program. I knew that time was short, so she reluctantly said she would ride along. When we got to the hospital where Dr. Mike's offices are, Alyce decided to wait in the car. I agreed because I foolishly thought it would be a quick appointment. Alyce doesn't go many places without a book, and I pictured her sitting in our locked car in Dr. Mike's very secure parking lot, reading. There was no reason to be worried; this is Green Bay, for heaven's sake, and I had left my cell phone with her. Alyce was two months short of fourteen, babysitter-trained, and smart as a whip. She was going to be fine. Yet for some reason, I needed right then to be sure. I asked to use the phone in the waiting area.

"Alyce, honey, I'm not done yet. This is taking longer than I thought. Why don't you come into the hospital and wait for me on the first floor? Just grab a seat and keep reading. I'll be right there."

Super. I probably have breast cancer, and my daughter will be waiting downstairs for me to drive us home. And I have to act as if everything is just fine.

What I had told Alyce was right. I was not finished. Dr. Mike read my films and ordered Step Three: a needle core biopsy. I walked down the hall to the ultrasound room with my gown flapping out to the sides. Little did I know that wearing a hospital gown was going to become commonplace for me. I was shown a dark room where another technician had me lie down on a table. She asked if she could hold my hand. I smiled. Right then, it seemed as if this woman, whom I had never met, had read my mind. I was scared and she knew it.

Handling the ultrasound wand deftly, she grazed over the lump. I asked her what she was looking for. She showed me two black blobs but said nothing else. *The explaining must be left to the doctor.* However, even with an untrained eye, it looked as if those two black blobs should not be there.

Once the suspicious areas had been located, the needle core biopsy was next. This test is NOT fun. It involves using a hollow "core" needle to remove small samples of breast tissue. Using the ultrasound as a guide, the doctor inserted the needle into the lump and removed a small bit of tissue. One click for each sample. *Click, click, click.* I can hear that clicking sound like it was yesterday.

Let me say this clearly: this procedure is painful. And with all of those fearful thoughts running through your head, it hurts even more. But I knew I would not be lying there, and Dr. Mike would not be doing this, if the situation were not serious. *So just breathe and let them take their samples.* After the tests were finally over, I was informed that it would be two days before the results would come back from the lab. TWO DAYS! It's a cruel aspect of modern medicine, but it's nobody's fault. They take their tests, and they send you home to wonder and worry.

I deserve an Academy Award for what happened next. I acted as if nothing was wrong when I went down to the first floor to pick up my patient, unworried daughter. "Just a minute, Mom. Let me finish this chapter. This book is so-o-o good," Alyce said, not taking her eyes off the printed page.

I smiled and sat down beside her while she read. An old expression came to mind: *ignorance is bliss.* Alyce looked so happy, so safe inside the imaginary world created by the author of a book she could not put down. She had no way of knowing about the band-aid on my right breast and the small ice pack in my bra. But I could not deceive myself. I knew full well this day was going to change my life forever. I could feel it in my bones.

Chapter 3

Bad News is Bad News

*What lies behind us and what lies before us
are tiny matters compared to what lies within us.*
Ralph Waldo Emerson

Dr. Mike called two days after the biopsy. As I said before, we go back a long way so we usually kid around a little when he phones. Not that day. He got straight to the point. "I have the results of your tests, Anita. It's bad news. The biopsy shows two malignant tumors called invasive adenocarcinoma. It's an aggressive form of cancer that needs to be taken care of immediately. But the good news is the odds are definitely in your favor."

I must have responded, but for the life of me, I cannot recall a single word I said. I do remember that after I hung up, I walked outside and stood in the middle of our manicured front lawn. Tony had just cut the grass and the lawnmower lines were visible; perfectly straight as always. It was an absolutely gorgeous summer day. The sun was shining gloriously overhead; there wasn't a cloud in the blue, crystal-clear Northeastern Wisconsin sky. I could smell the new-mown grass underfoot.

I just stood there, shaking my head in disbelief. "There must be some mistake," I reassured myself by speaking my thoughts aloud. "I simply cannot have cancer on a beautiful day like this."

I sat down on the steps of the front porch, trying to get my bearings. *But I trust Dr. Mike with my life, literally. He just said that I have breast cancer…so now what?* With that stark realization, I got up. My knees buckled, and I stumbled into the house. There was a tear running down my face, but I do not remember crying. My hands were shaking. My mind reeled, but not with fearful thoughts like: *How am I going to beat this? Will I lose my hair? Will Ray still love me? Am I going to die?* No, the all-consuming question in my mind was, *HOW am I going to tell my mother?*

Chapter 4

Your Fate Is in Your Genes

*Fear grows in darkness; if you think
there's a bogeyman around, turn on the light.*
Dorothy Thompson

Mom has always been a worrier. Always. She is one of those delightfully imaginative people who think bad things happen in direct proportion to how much you worry about them…in other words, the more you worry, the fewer bad things will happen. So it stands to reason that she especially excelled at worrying that something bad was going to happen to her children.

With my sister Colleen and me, she worried most about breast cancer. As I said earlier, breast cancer had claimed my maternal grandmother Evelyn at the age of 45. Mom was only eight years old at the time of her mother's death, so of course, just the word *cancer* terrified her. She always feared this "cancer-thing" would leave her children motherless, just as it had done to her. I was afraid of how she'd react to the news that I too had been stricken; I was specifically concerned that Mom might think this was all her fault.

Quite honestly, I did somehow always know I would have breast cancer. Always. Details were sketchy, but I knew my grandmother Evelyn found a lump and was diagnosed with cancer of the breast in 1952. Grandma Evelyn underwent radical surgery that led to a brief remission. But when severe hip pain and headaches sent her back to the doctor in 1954, tests confirmed new malignancies; the cancer had come back with a vengeance. It had metastasized into her bones and brain; nothing more could be done. She died at the age of 45 on October 5, 1954, when Mom was in third grade.

Grandma Evelyn was too young to die. My mom was too young to be without a mother. As I said, extensive information about Grandma Evelyn's battle was not available, but I knew this much—the danger of breast cancer was lurking in the shadows. It seemed as if it was just a matter of time. I could run, but I could not hide. So as much as we wished otherwise, my mother's nightmare and mine became reality. Dr. Mike's phone call would begin my personal journey, one that would take me to the edge of despair, of hell, and back, leaving me breastless, but still breathing.

Before I continue, I think it best to clear up any confusion about the cause of my disease. It was not anyone's fault. During chemotherapy, my doctors became convinced that something was going on genetically in my extended family. Since my grandmother, great-grandmother and great-great grandmother were all victims of breast cancer, and my Aunt Colette is a Stage 4 ovarian cancer survivor, a genetic counselor was commissioned to create a genetic profile. The results were most revealing.

After she mapped my family tree showing the high incidence of cancer in our family, the genetic counselor insisted I be tested for the BRCA1 mutation. A woman has up to an 85% chance of developing breast cancer in her lifetime if her BRCA1 gene, which is located on the "long arm" of chromosome 17, is abnormal. Considering my background, my doctors thought I might be carrying the mutation.

All it took was a simple blood test. The results were mixed. I do not have the mutated BRCA1 gene, but my test report indicated I do have another mutation on that chromosome called variant R496H. This abnormality in chromosome 17 is not definitively linked to breast cancer, but it is still a cause for concern. Perhaps research will someday conclude that this mutation is indeed a "breast cancer" precursor. I have a hard time believing that it is not linked somehow. *But for now, I must play the cards that I am dealt, BRCA1 or not,* I thought. *I will spend my energy fighting the disease, not cursing my genes.*

Both my Aunt Colette (the ovarian cancer survivor) and my sister agreed to be tested. Results showed Aunt Colette has the same mutation I do. That means the genetic defect came through my mother's side of the family. Mom and Aunt Colette must have received it from Grandma Evelyn, and I received it from my mother. Thankfully, Colleen does not have the mutated gene. When Alyce is in her thirties, she will probably want to be tested. Hopefully by that time, breast cancer will be a totally preventable disease of the past, like small pox or polio.

In the meantime, the ultimate purpose of genetic testing is to be proactive, to thwart the disease by early detection, thereby eliminating the element of surprise. For me, it was too late for that. My diagnosis was behind me. *Besides, the cure for cancer is probably decades away, I have to concentrate on beating this beast right now.* With my family history, and way before I found out about "genetic mutation," I knew that cancer was going to get me some day. I just never thought it would be so soon.

Chapter 5

Ray Can Fix Anything ... But This?

Informing family and friends that you have been diagnosed with breast cancer is NOT easy. Of course, I told my husband first. During the two days we had waited for the biopsy results, Ray and I had some heart-to-heart discussions. I admitted that I was scared, that I had been fortunate when the lump I had biopsied a couple years earlier turned out to be benign. I told him this time I was pretty sure it wouldn't be such good news.

Trying valiantly to digest Dr. Mike's bad news, I grabbed the phone and walked back outside. I needed fresh air, but it seemed as if I could not catch my breath. As I stood in the front yard, I fought hard to get a grip on myself. I knew Ray was anxiously awaiting my call, so I took a deep breath and dialed his number. Ray picked up his phone on the first ring. When I told him that the lump WAS cancer, he didn't say anything. At first I thought we had lost the connection. "Ray, honey…"

Ray has always been my rock and he certainly was that day. I could tell that he was shaken, but he said firmly, with a conviction that made me believe too, "No fear honey. We will come through this. I guarantee." That's my Ray.

Raphael Joseph Hockers. I do love that man. I met Ray the fall of my freshman year at Ashwaubenon High School. Ray walked into homeroom and smiled at me. I guess you could say it was the beginning of a love story that will never end. Ray and I were best friends first, then dated on and off during high school. It was nothing that serious romantically, just a wonderful time hanging out with each other and our friends.

Ray and I agree; we would not change a minute of our years at Ashwaubenon High. We occasionally run across people who say that they would never go back, never in a million years, but our time there was filled with good memories and wonderful people. We graduated in 1982 and went our separate ways. We were still good friends, just not boyfriend/girlfriend. We know now we each had to discover what else was out there.

During the next four years, Ray and I kept in casual contact, but somehow never connected. In my heart of hearts, I knew we cared for each other, even though we weren't "together." And it sure didn't help my dating prospects that I compared every man I went out with to Ray.

Then in 1986, from out of the blue, Ray called to invite me to join him for a drink. He was working at his family brick and tile business; I was attending classes at UW–Green Bay, working part-time, too busy to think about my high school best friend Ray. But I was just so pleased to hear from him that I made time to accept his invitation. We've been together ever since.

One year later, Ray proposed to me in front of his entire family at a family get-together. Thinking back now, it was not exactly the most romantic of places, but I was quick to say yes, and the planning of the first wedding in the DuJardin household began.

About six months before we were married, Ray and I bought the cutest stone house on a quaint street in Green Bay. It was small, only about 1000 square feet, but we loved it and every possibility that went along with owning our own place. The price tag? A whopping $48,000. We laugh now when we think you could ever buy a *house* for that amount. People pay more than that for a *car* today. But in 1987, we considered $48,000 a small fortune. No matter, we took the financial plunge. It was not a mistake. It was the perfect first home.

Even in his teens, Ray was a jack-of-all-trades. That man can fix anything. Literally. Ray grew up in the construction business, and recreation meant hanging out with your brothers at the brickyard on the weekend, getting dirty and greasy while fixing or building something. In the process, he learned more from his father and brothers than a trade school could ever teach. When it was time to remodel his very first house, Ray was ready for the challenge. The summer before we were married he spent every spare minute on our little stone house on McCormick Street. Hard work and sweat made that house our treasure.

We were married in November 1987. We had the typical 1980's wedding. The attire was big sleeves and big hair. The dinner was all-you-can-eat chicken served family style at one of the nicer local supper clubs. We had available our favorite beer on tap and any type of cocktail our guests could want. It was the kind of wedding that any couple in Green Bay dreamed of back then. Looking back, just like high school, we would not change a thing, especially moving into that cozy, comfy home on McCormick Street right after our honeymoon.

When we were blessed with Alyce and Tony, we brought our babies back to our little stone house. It was there they learned to ride their bikes, play in the sandbox, and run around like crazy little people. Because of that little stone house, we had a bank account, and we did not have car payments. Because of that little stone house, Ray was able to build our cottage in Door County. I have heard economists say that home ownership is the best way to get your own little piece of the American dream. We were living proof.

After seventeen happy years on McCormick Street, we came down with the "gotta have a bigger house" virus. Ray had always thought he should provide us with a bigger home. The kids were getting older, and even though we all loved the little stone house, they hinted that they needed more privacy. So did we. We had finally out-grown our first house; it was time to find a new home.

There are five tree-lined streets in Green Bay that I have always loved: St. Mary's Boulevard, Arrowhead Drive,

St. Francis Drive, Briar Lane, and Roselawn Boulevard. It may sound silly, but I always dreamed of living on one of them. I faithfully drove down those five streets for about two years, waiting for a realty sign to crop up in the front yard of the perfect house. However, every time I did spot a "For Sale" sign, the house seemed either too expensive or not the right fit.

While weekending at our place in Door County in February 2004, Ray and I stopped by a local tavern. As fate would have it, we struck up a conversation with a couple that lived near our cottage. We talked about the weather and the water and the crazy prices of real estate in Door County. We also mentioned we were looking for a bigger house in Green Bay.

For some reason, I told them about my five favorite streets. They both chimed in that his parents had a house on Arrowhead Drive. It had been empty for two years because his father had passed away and his mother was living with her daughter. He said they were thinking of listing the home in the near future.

I could not contain myself. "Would you let us see it before you sign with a realtor?"

"Sure, no problem. But let me warn you, it needs a lot of work. A LOT of work!"

"Like what?" I could see Ray's eyes lighting up like they always do when he sees an opportunity to make a good deal.

"Well, it's over forty years old…and it has never been remodeled…"

"That's actually a plus," Ray's voice rose slightly with excitement as it does when he is faced with an especially intriguing challenge. "You cannot believe how hard it can be to fix some do-it-yourselfer's botched job," he added.

"I see your point," the man said with a wry grin. "Not to worry. My parents weren't big on change."

"Hardly ever even rearranged the furniture," the wife chimed in. I couldn't help but see that our new acquaintances were apparently starting to think the same thing we were.

"Any idea of the price range?" I said, trying to be coy. I knew better than to be too eager, that if we were it was going to cost us a lot more money.

"We haven't really given it much thought..."

"Here," I wrote down our phone number on a cocktail napkin and handed it to him. "Seriously, call us before you list the house. Please?"

"No problem," he said, handing the napkin to his wife who folded it and put it in her pocket.

The rest, as they say, is "history." We were thrilled when he called, thrilled when we made the deal, thrilled when we signed the papers that made it all ours.

Believe me, he was not underestimating the condition of the house. But it was just what we were looking for: a big house in an established neighborhood. It was a two-story on a tree-lined street, and best of all, the kids could stay in their current schools. A major plus was that no one had done anything to the house in 42 years. Except for a few coats of paint, the house had not been touched. This ruled out the pitfalls of a "bad remodeling job" that Ray would have to "un-do" or "re-do."

Ray loves that kind of challenge. He smiled and chatted excitedly while we walked through the house. Knowing full well that he had to be brought back down to earth, I pointed out every single negative thing I could. He rebuffed every one of my objections with, "I can fix that." He was excited, but I was nervous as hell. I decided to put aside my fears and let myself get caught up in Ray's enthusiasm. We signed the papers and closed on May 28, 2004.

Fortunately, or rather unfortunately, we listed and sold our house on McCormick Street in two days. We asked the buyers if we might rent from them for two months so that we could try to pull off one huge remodeling job. They agreed and the "extreme makeover" began.

It was grueling. We worked our regular jobs all day, fed the kids, then headed off to the new house to work. We gutted the house…completely. Seven full dumpsters later, no room was left untouched. Ray re-worked the floor plan, framed in new rooms, and added special touches as we went along to make it fit our family's needs. We hired sub-contractors: electricians, plasterers, masons, plumbers, heating and air conditioning experts. All worked their magic, but there was still so much for us to do. Ray was exhausted but absolutely pleased with the progress we were making.

As I said, Ray can fix just about anything; and if he doesn't know how, he's not afraid to ask. He touched base with his friends in the building business and made sure that everything he was doing made sense. He worked like a dog those two months and turned the old house into a beautiful, contemporary home. Eight weeks had seemed like an eternity when we made the deal with the new owners of our old house, but flew by when it came right down to it. We finished just in time to meet our closing date. We said our good-byes to McCormick Street and moved into our dream home on August 1. We could not believe our good fortune. This was the house we had always dreamed of. The kids were happy, we were ecstatic; our little family of four was on top of the world. It was perfect. Thirteen days after moving in, I found the lump. Perfect, my ass.

Chapter 6

A Shoulder to Lean On

*No matter how dark things seem to be or actually are, raise your sights
and see the possibilities—they're always there.*
Norman Peale

Was it divine intervention or just a cruel twist of fate?
Whichever it was, the day Dr. Mike delivered the bad news, I
was standing out in the middle of the front yard, still talking
to Ray, when my parents pulled into the driveway. They had
taken the kids for the day, and Alyce and Tony waved to me
from the back seat as Dad parked the car. With not a care in
the world, the kids ran right past me into the house. Their
only worry was who was going to get to their favorite
computer video game first. *To be a kid again…*

Motioning to Mom and Dad to stay outside, I told Ray that
I loved him and clicked the off-button on the cordless. As
Mom remembers, my hands were shaking and she knew
something was wrong. Really wrong. There was not going to
be an easy way to tell them, so I said flat out, "Mom, Dad, I
have breast cancer."

In shock and grief that her worst nightmare was coming
true, Mom blinked hard and a look of absolute horror came
over her face. She doubled over, right there in the driveway.
Dad shook his head in disbelief, then went over to put his arm

around Mom. She straightened herself and leaned against the hood of the car. I just stood there, dumbfounded and in shock myself. It was like a tear-jerker scene in a sappy chick flick. But this wasn't a movie. This was for real. This was my *life,* and *we* were embarking on the ride of our lives. We might have been physically prepared for this cancer-thing, but not mentally.

To be sure, I am strong and confident, traits I inherited from my mother. I have always been strong; opinionated, in charge; okay, okay...I am Anita. I control situations, but right from the start, we all knew there was no controlling this. Still, I couldn't let that matter. That day and every day since, I have tried to stay as strong as I can, for my entire family, but especially for my mother. I have to show her that this beast can be conquered, that I will not die like her mother did.

Of course, I could have fought for my life against this monstrous disease without Mom. I could have because I would have had no choice. I have a husband and two children who need me. Ray was right beside me, as always, and my friends were too. But, thank God, Mom was there, loving and supporting me in ways only a mother can, providing her sweet reassurance that no matter what, I was not going to have to do this alone.

Chapter 7
To Be a Kid Again

There is more inside you than you dare think.
David Brower

Anita Marie DuJardin was born on March 14, 1964, the oldest of four children, to two young high school sweethearts. They were and still are very much in love. I have always believed that we are a very close family because of them. Mom and Dad's love was so strong for each other that it rubbed off on us.

Exactly one year and one week after I was born, along came my brother, Jon. Matthew joined the brood three years later. Our comfortable family of five was going about its business, living a normal, peaceful life until the autumn of 1972 when our parents threw us all a curve ball.

We were at the dinner table that evening when my Dad announced, "Well, kids, there's going to be a surprise in this house."

Now, you may find this totally ridiculous, because it is, but Jon and I looked at each other in panic. "No way! We're getting a dog!" I whispered to Jon. I am not really sure why, but I cannot remember ever really liking or feeling comfortable around dogs. It sounds silly, but it was a big deal for me at the time. I could not believe it. My parents were springing another dog on us!

Mom and Dad had tried the "dog-thing" before. Dad would bring a puppy home. That little fur-ball would be maybe six inches off the ground, but Jon and I were so petrified of dogs that we would act like absolute idiots. We would sit on the swings in the backyard with our legs hiked up. We would stand behind the railing on the porch in a futile attempt to put a barrier between us and the poor little dog. As if this precious little thing could harm us! But childish fears trumped even the most intense puppy love. Eventually the puppy would be sent to greener, more hospitable pastures inhabited by children who would appreciate it.

So it was that evening, that no matter how cute the puppy in question was going to be, Jon and I would have none of it. The lone dissenter was Matt. "Dogs are the coolest!" he chirped.

"You're only four," Jon objected. "You think everything's the coolest."

Then Mom started to laugh. Jon and I could not see the humor in the situation at all. This was not, in our opinion, a laughing matter. I honestly remember sitting at the kitchen table, glaring at my mother. But I needn't have been so spiteful; there would be no dog. No dog, but the "surprise" was potentially much, much worse. We were going to have a baby.

I was only eight years old, but I began to pray immediately. It was hard enough living with two brothers. I could not, would not, live with three. "Please, God," I begged, "don't let it be a boy. If it is, I might just be the youngest girl ever to run away and join the circus."

Chapter 8
My Shining Light

I've heard it said that people come into our lives for a reason,
bringing something we must learn and we are led to those who
help us most to grow, if we let them, and we help them in return.
Well, I don't know if I believe that's true, but I know I'm
who I am today because I knew you.
Glinda in "Wicked"

I am quite sure that most people do not remember what they were doing on April 10, 1973, but believe me, I do. That day I was doing my best to sell myself to Grandma Millie. I believed God would hear my prayer for a sister, but just in case, I would turn to my grandmother for deliverance. I was determined to live with her if this new baby was a boy. There was no doubt in my mind. Just surviving the teasing that two brothers can lay on you is hard enough, but now there was the distinct possibility I might have three.

At that time, fathers were just beginning to be allowed into the delivery room. My dad said he was *not* interested. He promised to be at the hospital to hand out the cigars, but not in the delivery room. As fate would have it, Dad was scheduled for a one-day business trip the day Mom went into labor. Using a pre-arranged "just-in-case" maneuver, Mom called a neighbor lady to drive her to the hospital, to have my

SISTER, of course. Then Mom called my Grandma to pick us up. My brothers, who were positive that another little brother was soon to arrive into the nest, were beaming. If looks could kill, my brothers would have seen their obnoxious little lives cut short that very moment.

I do not remember the ride to Grandma's. I was probably in a trance, doing meditation, praying that God would listen. I do remember being nervously perched on Grandma's davenport. (Remember when they used to call a couch the "davenport"?) My brothers were relentless. Up to their old tricks, they were skipping around the living room, singing, "It's gonna be a boy. It's gonna be a boy...what should we name him?" Being the "dirty looks" queen at the time, I made the nastiest faces I could at them, but it didn't work.

Grandma must have known how nervous I was because she recruited me to sit by the phone in case the hospital called. I stared and stared at that telephone, sometimes thinking I could make it ring, then hoping it wouldn't because I was afraid of what the news might be. It took forever, and when the phone finally rang, my heart stopped.

I quickly went over the plan in my mind. *Grab the suitcase, load up my stuff, beg Grandma to take me in.* Grandma answered the phone, leaning on the counter, holding the old-fashioned green phone with the very short cord up to her ear. There was a twinkle in her eye when she looked right at me and said, "Wonderful, I am so glad IT's healthy..."

Tears welled up in my eyes, and then she had mercy on me. She whispered, "Anita, Colleen is here." Thank Goodness! I could go home. There need be no new life at Grandma Millie's for me. I had a baby sister. And what's more, Colleen was mine and the boys would not be touching her.

I have heard horror stories about sisters who do not get along. That is totally incomprehensible to me. As I said earlier, I was nine when Colleen was born. That made me the perfect age to have a baby sister. I put my fully-developed "Mom Jr." skills to use immediately. As far as I was concerned, Colleen was my baby, a living baby doll that was all mine. I was so protective of that little girl. I put her in my doll crib; I wrapped her in my doll blankets; I "fed" her the fake food from my make-believe doll kitchen. I cranked the baby swing when it stopped rocking, and she seemed to be permanently attached to my hip. She was so little, and she was so cute.

Those first five years passed as if female sibling rivalry is a myth invented by psychologists pushing self-help books. I celebrated turning ten about the time Colleen took her first steps. How could you resist her? She made the cutest faces, and when she started talking, I sometimes laughed so hard I cried at her silly pronunciations. I played board games with her, read her books, and helped her learn to tie her shoes. I am sure I was a huge help to my mother who also had my two rambunctious brothers underfoot. All the time I spent with Colleen must have given Mom an occasional moment to get some housework done. Lord knows, the cooking, the cleaning, and the laundry for four children never seemed to end. Of course, it also bonded my sister to me in ways that would be demonstrated over and over again during our adult lives and with my ordeal decades later with the beast called cancer. I cannot imagine surviving during those dreadful days of treatment and recovery if Colleen had not been there.

Looking back, there were a couple of times when Colleen and I weren't close: my high school years and her college years. I started my first year of high school the same year Colleen entered kindergarten. I was a typical freshman, and she was a normal five-year-old. It was inevitable that the generation gap would set in. She was not so cute anymore; it seemed as if there were light years between us. She was always in my stuff. She was always asking questions. She was always looking for me…basically driving the self-absorbed teenager I was back then absolutely crazy. So it stands to reason that a hard-working student with a busy social life would have no time or interest in being a "Mom Jr." to her little sister.

Suffice it to say Colleen and I somehow muddled through my high school years, but we did have our moments. I tried out for cheerleading at Ashwaubenon High School my junior year. In the 1980s, all you needed was a set of lungs and a smile. I had both and was not afraid to use them. I earned a spot on the varsity squad, and I took to cheerleading like a fish to water. I was loud. Really loud. I loved getting the crowd revved up, not to mention thinking I looked sort of cute in my uniform. I loved everything about being a cheerleader: pep rallies, making posters, football games, and my personal favorite, wrestling matches.

People who know me know that I love to lead. I admit, with no hesitation, that I like to be in charge. It is something

I do really well. So of course, "cheerleading and Anita" went together like cake and ice cream. Colleen enjoyed the games and wrestling matches, watching her big sister and wishing she could wear my uniform. I would smile and wink to Colleen in the stands, and she would beam. She obviously thought her big sister was something pretty special.

I left for college in the Fall of 1982 to attend the University of Wisconsin in Madison. Colleen was nine and in third grade, the same age I was when she had come into my life. College was so exciting: new challenges, new people, new me…I wanted to experience it all. I was so caught up in my own "leaving the nest" that I did not realize just how lost my sister was without me. I can recall Mom, Dad and Colleen helping me move into my cramped dormitory room in Sellery Hall. I was so excited about being on my own that I never gave a thought as to how Colleen might feel. I do remember her looking at the floor a lot that day and hugging me for a long time. Mom told me the ride home from Madison was long for Colleen and that she had tried to hide her tears, but could not.

I realized later how hard that must have been on a nine-year-old. The person you have lived with all your life, clung to, looked up to, was leaving, moving far away to a little room in a very tall building. But I was too full of myself to think of Colleen.

However, our separation did not last long. I quickly found out that I am a complete homebody, most comfortable in familiar, safe surroundings. I was not happy being three hours away from my family. In January 1984, after three semesters at

UW–Madison, I transferred to the University of Wisconsin–Green Bay campus. I was back home.

During my remaining college years, I lived at home, and Colleen and I reconnected. The only other time that we lost a bit of contact was when Colleen left for college. She was trying to pave a new road for herself, just as I had done. I was a new mother to my daughter Alyce at the time, and our lives could not have been further apart. But again, we reconnected to make it back to the relationship that started from day one…the love of two sisters. To this day there are no two sisters, anywhere, that are closer than we are.

Naturally, the news of my breast cancer devastated Colleen. When I called her at her office in Chicago, she was incredulous. I remember telling her straight out. "Colleen, I don't know how to tell you this, but I have breast cancer." There was absolute disbelief in her voice. This could not be happening to her big sister.

Then, for a long moment, we both said nothing. But I knew she was still there, and in that silence, I swear I heard her thinking. *"We will beat this, Anita. Whatever you need. Whatever it takes."* That "whatever" would take me to places no human being should ever have to go. But I went, I endured, and I came back. And Colleen was there every step of the way. The entire time I was fighting breast cancer, Colleen was there at my side. Her love, a sister's love, was a shining light during some very dark days.

Chapter 9
Sleep, Eat and Cry

Hope is the thing with feathers...that perches in the soul...and sings
the tune without the words...and never stops...at all.
Emily Dickinson

After I told my family, I called Dr. Mike back. It took us a minute or two to gather our thoughts; then we formulated a plan. He suggested we make an appointment with a local breast surgeon named Dr. Colette. How we got this incredibly talented woman in little Green Bay, Wisconsin, is beyond me. But remember, there are no accidents; she must have been on my path. "One wrinkle," he said, "unfortunately Dr. Colette's on vacation, which means you'll have to wait five days to see her."

Five days is an eternity when you know there's something growing inside of you that is hell-bent on killing you. You want it GONE, like RIGHT NOW! Dr. Mike knew that I was a nervous wreck, who wouldn't be, so he gave us another option. We could go to Chicago where he knew other excellent cancer specialists. He said he could set up the appointments, even brief the doctors on my case, but he really urged me to wait for Dr. Colette.

Ray and I both wondered if delaying things might be a fatal mistake. "Is there time to wait, Dr Mike?" I asked.

"Absolutely, Anita. And if you were MY wife, I would tell you the same thing. Wait for Dr. Colette." So we waited. But as you can imagine, that was a very long five days.

Mom and Colleen went with me to my first consultation with Dr. Colette. Dr. Mike had booked the appointment for 8:30 a.m., the earliest available. As it turned out, this was a huge conflict for Ray because he was needed at work that morning for a very important meeting. "It's like being stuck between a rock and a hard place, honey," he said when he told me. I could tell how desperately he wanted to be with me, but I also knew how much his boss was counting on him. At the time, we had no way of knowing this would be just the beginning of Ray being torn between his work, our kids, and my illness.

I told him not to worry, that Mom and Colleen would be there, that it was "girl" stuff anyway. It took a lot of persuading, but I finally convinced him he would be with me in my heart. So on that fateful morning, I kissed and hugged him several times and sent him off to work. A few minutes later, I hugged and kissed my kids, heaved a sigh of resignation, and left our dream house to begin my journey into hell.

Within the hour, Mom, Colleen and I were seated in Dr. Colette's consultation room. We had no idea what to expect, but we knew the moment we met her that Dr. Mike had not steered us in the wrong direction. She came into the room wearing scrubs and a pair of running shoes. There was a smile on her face and a bounce in her step. She did not mince words, explaining that I did not do anything wrong to "bring on" breast cancer. Dr. Colette explained that nobody knows for sure why the tumors started growing. Maybe it was the right day, maybe the moon was rising or the stars were aligned at just the right angle. *Maybe it was on my path. Does it really matter why? No; it's neither here nor there. What we need now is to concentrate on stopping it.*

A friendly, efficient and empathetic woman, Dr. Colette quickly outlined her suggested course of treatment. Because of the aggressive nature of my cancer, she wanted me to start neoadjuvant chemotherapy. In layman's terms, this means a patient has chemotherapy first, then surgery. This is opposite of everything that we have come to regard as the "usual and customary" sequence of treatment for malignancies.

"Anita, your test results indicate you have at least two tumors in your right breast," she said, explaining the reasoning behind this do-things-in-reverse strategy. She looked me straight in the eye, gave me another of her magnificent smiles, and went on. "I know all cancer patients want their tumors out immediately, and I completely understand that." Determined to be brave, but fighting back tears, I managed only a nod.

"Of course, this is your body, and I will proceed any way you choose…but here's how I look at it." All three of us listened intently as she continued.

"Neoadjuvant chemotherapy attacks the cancer while it's still there. If you have the surgery first, we can't see the tumors shrinking. So how are we to know if the chemotherapy is working or not?" We discussed Dr. Colette's point of view for a bit while she listened patiently. Though they didn't come right out and say it, I could tell Mom and Colleen tended to agree with her. It made sense to me too, but I couldn't resist saying, "We all know people with cancer, Doctor. And they all had surgery first."

Dr. Colette pulled out a writing tablet, took a pen from her pocket, and began to sketch. "I think it will be easier for you to understand if you let me show you what cancer looks like," she said as she drew pictures of breasts with tumors in them.

My hand was shaking as she handed me the notepad. I stared at the drawing in silence. "Nasty," was all that finally came out of my mouth. I showed Mom the drawing. She studied it a moment, then put on her "brave" face and passed the picture to Colleen who just nodded, fighting valiantly to hold back her tears.

"And this is what a cancer cell looks like," Dr. Colette said, taking the tablet from Colleen and drawing another picture. She was a pretty good artist and had obviously done this before.

The shock was lessening; I was starting to feel like my old self again. "So those are the little bastards that want me dead," I quipped.

We all laughed and the tension was broken.

"Again, I will proceed any way you choose," she replied. "But my recommendation for you is neoadjuvant chemotherapy." She was the professional. Who was I to disagree? I looked at Mom, at Colleen, at the doctor in whose hands I was entrusting my life. Neoadjuvant chemotherapy was my choice.

Dr. Colette took the notepad once again, turned the page, jotted down four words, and handed it to me. She had written *You* at the top of the page and below it, *Sleep, Eat* and *Cry.*

"I need three things from you. I need you to get your sleep, 8 hours a day. I need you to eat; this is not the time to start a diet. You must keep up your strength. And thirdly, I want you to cry."

Incredulous, I stared blankly at Dr. Colette. *Cry? What are you talking about?*

"Anita, you need to cry. If you cry too much, call me. If you don't cry at all, call me. But if you cry once in awhile, that's good. You are human and this is frightening."

I swallowed hard and nodded my head in agreement. "Okay, then," I decided. "That's what I'll do. So what comes next?"

"Let me take a look." She began a thorough examination of both of my breasts. I closed my eyes and prayed. *Please, God. I'm begging now. Please let her say this is all a mistake, that I do NOT have cancer at all.* I was prepared to go home, to go on living my life, taking my health for granted. But all my hopes were dashed, my pretty dreams shattered when she said, "I'm sure there are at least two, maybe even three tumors, Anita. I want to do another needle core biopsy to be sure."

This time when I looked at the ultrasound, my newly-trained eye saw that the third suspicious area meant trouble. There were now three fast growing tumors in my breast. Had another one sprouted the week while I waited? Or were my breasts so dense that the first ultrasound picked up only two? Such thoughts were a useless waste of time. I needed all my energy to deal with the prospect that this merciless disease was my mortal enemy bent on destroying me. There was only one thing to do: confront my illness head on.

And confront it I did. I was not happy about it, but I immediately agreed to have a sentinel node biopsy the following Monday. This procedure would tell us if the cancer had spread to the lymph nodes. "It will help matters greatly if the cancer is contained to the breast," Dr. Colette said hopefully. *Damn right! It'll help a lot. Dear God, please, don't let it be in my lymph nodes.*

Chapter 10
Two Boobs or Not Two Boobs...

A bend in the road is not the end of the road,
unless you refuse to take the turn.
Anonymous

I have always said I would not undergo reconstruction if I lost a breast, to cancer or anything else. I did not, and do not, want anything artificial implanted into my body. Other women feel exactly the opposite. Please don't get me wrong. I respect any woman for whatever choice she makes about this highly sensitive and subjective decision. But for me, I was quite certain that reconstruction was out of the question. Since I was never a big fan of my own boobs, I could not imagine having fake ones. However, with push coming to shove, I thought I should at least cover all the bases and visit a plastic surgeon.

I admit I am an incorrigible people-watcher, and that day, as I sat in the waiting area, I studied the faces of the women who came out of the examining rooms' doorway. It was all I could do to stop myself. I wanted to approach each and every one of them and ask, "Did you have cancer? Did you decide for or against reconstruction? How did you decide what to do?"

Here I had thought my mind was completely made up, and now I suddenly wanted, no, desperately needed, to talk to someone who was more experienced about this. But I couldn't get up the courage to ask anyone, so I just sat there with my miserable thoughts.

Am I making the wrong decision? Am I being too stubborn about this? Every guy's a breast man...Ray said it's up to me, but would he really rather I did reconstruct? Guess I'll have to talk to the doctor; he must deal with this kind of indecision all the time.

I have to say the doctor really knew his stuff. He introduced me to silicone and saline implants. I shook my head. He enthusiastically suggested a tram flap procedure. He explained the operation involved removing an oval section of skin, fat, and muscle from the lower half of the abdomen. It is then moved up to the breast area through a tunnel which the surgeon creates under the skin. The tissue is then shaped into a natural-looking breast mound and sewn into place.

He was really persuasive. "Anita, this is also a great way to get a tummy tuck."

No thanks. I'm not opposed to a flatter stomach, but I think I'll just stick to sit-ups.

"However," he went on in a more cautionary tone as he noted my resistance, "if your surgery turns out to be a bilateral mastectomy, you probably don't have enough fat in your belly area to form TWO breast mounds."

Believe it or not, I do not remember vomiting even once in my entire life, but at that moment, I felt like I was going to throw up right there in his office. Just the term *breast mounds* made me physically sick.

"Now come on," I chirped in an attempt to quell the nausea rising from my stomach to my throat. "How about using some of the fat from my butt?" He ignored my failed attempt at humor. I said I would think about it. I did. For less than a minute. I knew in my gut that I had been right about reconstruction. It was not for me, and I was not going to do it. It was simple punctuation. Breast mounds. Question Mark. No thank you. Period. The fact that I was physically sick when I left his office. Exclamation point.

I called Dr. Mike's clinic the day after the plastic surgery consultation. This may sound ridiculous, but I wanted to see the pathology report for myself. Why…who knows? As if I was going to understand the medical jargon contained in a pathology report. But you grab at straws. You try anything, anything to make sense of the fact that you are locked in a life and death struggle with this monster called cancer. The receptionist said Dr. Mike would make time for me, whenever I got there.

I knew full well that Dr. Mike had not misread my test results. Perhaps I just needed to see him, to have him reassure me. I wanted him to tell me once again that everything was going to be all right. As always, he went the extra mile. He handed me the report; I started reading. *Hockers, Anita M. Right breast, needle core biopsy: invasive adenocarcinoma.*

There was more, but the rest was unreadable through my tears. How could a mere compilation of words, arranged and printed in ordinary black type on a simple white piece of paper, have the power to destroy me? But rock my world it did.

Dear man that he is, Dr. Mike just listened. I cried a little, then I got mad, then I cried harder. When he sensed I was finally ready to listen, he said what I had come to hear. "Anita, you are going to beat this. You are NOT going to die. You are going to be around for a long, long time." Then he gave me the biggest, most sincere hug I have ever received from someone to whom I am not related. Neither of us let go for what seemed like a very long time.

Chapter 11

Cocktails Anyone?

We could never learn to be brave and patient,
if there were only joy in the world.
Helen Keller

No woman should start her week with a sentinel node biopsy, but the following Monday there I was, being prepped for one. As I mentioned earlier, the sentinel node biopsy determines whether or not the cancer has spread. This node is the first lymph node in the armpit area that the breast drains to, hence the name *sentinel.* Every step of the way, I was told what would happen, as if that would somehow lessen the discomfort. It did not.

This is not a medical procedure; it could be compared to legalized torture. But there is no way around it. If the cancer is moving out of the breast, it will travel through the sentinel node first. It is crucial that it be located and tested in order for the doctors to successfully map out a patient's entire course of treatment.

Before this procedure was available, a surgeon had no idea which node was the sentinel. The doctor would have to guess and hope for the best. In an effort to err on the side of caution, several nodes would be removed and tested for cancer cells. If the results came back negative, it was assumed the malignancy had not spread. A patient would go home with the happy diagnosis that the lymph nodes were free of cancer.

However, because guessing was involved, at times the surgeon would not find the right node. The actual sentinel node was not found and therefore not tested. If this node did have cancer, the disease could recur. As you can see, it is therefore absolutely essential that this sentinel node, or as some people call it, the "guardian angel node," be located and tested. If not, it can spell major trouble for the patient.

To find the sentinel node, the doctor injects a radioactive substance called a tracer into the ducts of the breast. This is the difficult and painful part because the tracer must be injected into the sensitive nipple area by means of a fine needle. They use a local anesthetic, but it hurts like hell. Trust me. Four injections to the nipple will bring tears to anyone's eyes.

On the flip side, the procedure is really quite interesting. As the test progressed, I could watch the radioactive dye on the monitor travel through my right breast. I stared in utter fascination as it trailed out toward my armpit, searching for the sentinel node. Then suddenly, there it was, glowing hottest radioactively. It was the one Dr. Colette was looking for, and it "lit up" on the screen, as if it was indeed a warning signal of danger within.

This part of the procedure over, I was wheeled into surgery and put to sleep. (That was my favorite part). During surgery, Dr. Colette carefully removed the sentinel node and two nearby. Since I had decided on neoadjuvant chemotherapy, she also installed a "port-a-cath" which would enable the cancer-fighting chemicals to be dispensed directly into the main blood supply entering the heart. This facilitates the process so that chemotherapy can be quickly and efficiently delivered to all parts of the body. The port is roughly the size of a nickel, inserted directly beneath the skin about four inches below my collarbone. Having the port installed was a blessing. It saved my arms from the numerous pokes that would have been otherwise required during chemotherapy.

One thing that definitely helped me that day was that I had a visitor during the dye injection. Dr. Mike stopped by. He went out of his way, during his busy day, to come and hold my hand. What a guy. This procedure was agony, but the pain was lessened having Dr. Mike's hand to hold.

After the procedure, I was taken to the recovery area. I woke up slowly and smiled when I saw Ray. The rest of my family was waiting anxiously in a nearby room. I asked Ray if he had heard anything yet. He said Dr. Colette had dropped by to see them while I was in the recovery room. "She said the lymph nodes looked suspect," Ray reported, "but she also said not to get ahead of ourselves; that we'll know more after the pathology report comes back."

I went home with a very heavy heart. *How can things get any worse?* They did. That night I found out the hard way that I am allergic to the radioactive blue dye. I broke out in hives. They started at my toes and crept up my body. But it was nothing an antihistamine couldn't cure. Benadryl got the best of the hives in a few hours. If only antihistamines could do the same thing to cancer.

Two days later, Dr. Colette called to tell me the bad news: the cancer had indeed spread to the lymph nodes. "When the cancer exits the primary site through the lymph system, it spreads to other parts of the body," she told me.

I replied, my voice almost a whisper, "And that's why doctors say finding it early helps so much…" I remembered all the things I had done to facilitate early detection. *All the things that hadn't accomplished a damn thing.*

"Definitely. Finding the cancer before it spreads is important," she replied, "but, let me reassure you, Anita, there are many things we can do to stop your cancer in its tracks. The first thing we'll do is schedule an appointment for you to see an oncologist."

Oncologist. Great. I am now officially a "cancer patient." Wonderful. Malignant tumors are spreading their deathly tentacles throughout my body, and my life is now in the hands of strangers. I cannot believe this. I'm Anita, the super manager, the control freak, and I've lost the ability to control anything.

The very next day, Mom, Ray and I met Dr. J. As with Dr. Colette, I had no idea what to expect, but the man is everything an oncologist should be. Serious medical conditions like cancer make you feel tiny and insignificant, but when Dr. J walked into the room, he immediately made me feel important. He's an honest, determined man, with an intensely thoughtful demeanor. It's as if he's on a mission, and that day, thank God, his mission was to save my life.

He said his hellos and then focused on me. He did not take his eyes off me during our entire conversation. I was the patient, and it was as if to him nothing else mattered, as if there was no one else in the room. One of my favorite things is when people look you straight in the eye. It tells me that *I matter*. I trusted Dr. J immediately.

The last thing people in my shoes need is sugar-coating the truth. "This is not going to be easy, Anita," he explained. "Fighting cancer is difficult, but, if we fight hard enough and long enough, we can prevail."

My apprehension was dispelled as he continued to explain the course of therapy he was recommending. "Adriamycin and cytoxan for the first four rounds," he said. "We mix it, sort of like a cocktail."

"Good," I said mischievously. "I like cocktails, especially Limon and Diet Coke." My clumsy attempt at humor hit the mark, and we all laughed. It felt so good to laugh.

Then he grew serious again. "After that, we assess your progress. We'll do surgery if you aren't responding."

"Responding?"

"If the tumors aren't shrinking. But if they are, we follow with four rounds of Taxotere. It all depends on how stubborn your cancer is."

How do these medical miracle workers decide which drugs to use in each case? It's amazing. It seemed like everyone I talked to during my chemotherapy was on a different round of this or that. A different *cocktail* for each situation. I realize today that my course of treatment was pretty much standard, but it was "tweaked" to meet my own special needs, as it is for every other cancer patient.

Chemotherapy. A benign-sounding word. It falls off the tongue like aroma therapy or massage therapy. But there is no comparison. Chemotherapy is not benign; it is a draconian thing to do to the human body. As I mentioned earlier, during my sentinel node biopsy, Dr. Colette had installed a chemotherapy port in my chest to facilitate the injection of the anti-cancer drugs. I knew and yet I did not know what I was in for when I ended my consultation with Dr. J. I summoned up all my courage and left him with the words we both needed to hear. "Okay, Dr. J. You're on my team. I'm wired up," I said, pointing to my port, "and ready to go. Let's start fighting."

After we said our good-byes, Ray and I hurried out of the hospital and into the bright sunlight, trying to catch up with Mom who had said she needed "some fresh air." She had almost sprinted off the elevator. "More likely she needed to get out of this house of horrors," I told Ray. When we spotted her, we stopped, our hearts breaking. She stood alone in the parking lot, face to the heavens, her arms at her side.

After a few moments, Ray and I approached. Suddenly, I felt this horrible, sickening feeling in the pit of my stomach. It stopped me dead in my tracks. I fumbled, staggered, and grabbed my knees, unable to catch my breath. My body was shaking from the inside out.

"Anita, are you all right?" Ray said, his voice breaking as he grabbed my arm.

"I cannot have cancer, honey," I cried out. "I can't. What am I going to do? I just can't have cancer."

Her reverie broken by my uncharacteristic behavior, Mom came rushing to my side. Still leaning on Ray, I stood up and reached for her. Her facial expression was a mixture of grief and frustration. I knew exactly what she was thinking as we embraced. She could not fix this. She could not write a note and say that Anita was sick but she would be back in school tomorrow. She could not give me a couple aspirin and call me in the morning. By the look on her face, she could not comprehend how I could be this sick.

Neither could I, because I didn't feel sick. The truth is I've always been pretty healthy. I didn't need to see Dr. Mike, or any other doctor for that matter, very often. That's not to say I was unfamiliar with hospitals. Some time after my second pregnancy, I needed varicose vein removal. An ill-advised move in the sand during an intense volleyball game necessitated a right ACL repair. After tripping over the vacuum cleaner hose, I tore my rotator cuff, which had to be fixed if I planned on doing any more housecleaning. So I had some experience with what it took to go under the knife, what was involved in recovery, rehabilitation, and healing.

But as we stood huddled together in that parking lot, I knew with no uncertainty that those three surgeries were nothing compared to what I was about to endure. When I was in grade school, I read a magazine article about how fortune tellers use crystal balls to see into the future. I thought at the time that sounded really cool. Now I know that one of life's greatest blessings is that we cannot see into the future. Thank God that I couldn't foresee how my life would become a routine of consultations, tests, procedures, surgeries, recovery, and then more tests to see if the course of treatment was successful. You bet your butt it's a good thing I didn't have a crystal ball. If I had, I may have seriously considered throwing in the towel right then and there.

Chapter 12

The Cure Is a Killer

If you lose hope, somehow you lose the vitality that keeps life moving,
you lose that courage to be, that quality that helps you go on in
spite of it all. And so today I still have a dream…
Martin Luther King, Jr.

I need to state clearly, that right from the beginning, I did what I had to do because I had no choice. Well, that's not quite true. I have heard of some cancer victims who do not fight, so I suppose I could have just let the disease take its course. But I have a husband, two children, a close-knit family, a wide circle of friends and co-workers, all of them counting on me. And being Anita, once I decided to fight, I fought the cancer tooth and nail with every single weapon that modern medicine provides.

The next weapon happened to be a PET scan, a test I had the morning of my first day of chemotherapy. PET (Positron Emission Tomography) is used to determine if the cancer has spread beyond the initial site or sites to any other organs. PET scans are a form of what is called "nuclear" medicine and are really quite intriguing. The PET scan finds tumors by searching for "hot spots" in the body. Before he began, the technician sat me down and explained to me in detail how the scan would work.

"PET is like an MRI, but it's 3-D and in color. Malignant cells divide very quickly, and they use a lot of glucose in the process. That's sugar in a form the body can use. What we do is inject radioactive glucose into your veins. It circulates throughout your body and attaches itself to those rapidly-growing cells. The radiation then shows up on the scan, identifying where those abnormal cells reside...a hot spot."

"You mean cancer," I said. He nodded...I understood. For some reason, I immediately thought of one of those early video games, Pac Man.

This test was nothing compared to the sentinel node biopsy. It was almost boring. First, I was injected with the radioactive glucose, then instructed to wait for an hour in a dark room with NO stimulation. No reading, no lights, no sounds, no nothing. I was told that the reason my pre-procedure environment had to be totally sterile was because any stimulation to the brain might cause a "false positive" report. There was a chance that the radioactive glucose could attach itself to *activated* areas of the brain, seeming to indicate there was cancer present, even if there wasn't. In such a "clean" environment, I fell asleep and had to be awakened by the technician who came to transport me. I was placed in a cylinder, similar to an MRI machine, but shorter. The actual test took only about 20 minutes, after which I was released to my first round of chemotherapy.

I had heard horror stories about chemotherapy. It was like when we were in our twenties, friends would tell us about the horrors of childbirth. That being said, I was a little scared. A lot of what people told me turned out to be true, but everyone handles chemotherapy differently. Some patients get sick and throw up, some are so tired they cannot pick their heads up off the pillow, and some are just scared, scared to death.

I can honestly say that initially I was not afraid of chemotherapy. I am not sure why, but I looked at it as something that needed to be done. *There are no other options, so let's get down to business.* I suppose that up until that morning, I was still in denial. *Come on, not me. This cannot be cancer.* The only time that I really felt like a "cancer patient" was when I met with Dr. J. It's as if my subconscious had interpreted the situation as a simple medical issue.

Nevertheless, a month after I found that cursed lump, here I was, destined to join a room full of "cancer patients" to begin chemotherapy. All my denial disappeared when I walked into the hospital chemotherapy wing. It hit me like a ton of bricks. With unsteady steps, terrified by what being here meant, I desperately tried to push away my fearful thoughts. *If I walk into that room, if I mingle with those bald, sick people, if I sit down with "cancer patients," then I am one too.*

Thank heavens Ray, Mom, and Aunt Colette were there, or I might have run away. I looked at them and knew I had to stay. Aunt Colette had completed her chemotherapy just two years earlier for her Stage 4 ovarian cancer. She looked at me with eyes that only a cancer patient could understand. She knew how sick I was going to be; she had been there and now her niece was going, too. She put her hand on my shoulder, almost as if she was trying to send some of her strength my way. *She stared death straight in the eye; she's still here. I can do it too.* I smiled, and she knew my thoughts without me saying a single word.

The procedure began. As Dr. J had ordered, I would have four rounds, spaced two weeks apart, during which I would be given a mixture of adriamycin and cytoxan. It was to be the same each time. Let's tell it like it is. These medicines are hard core. The nurses dress in rubber gowns and rubber gloves because these chemicals will burn anything with which they come in contact. I was told that for the next 48 hours, every time I needed to use the toilet, I had to flush it TWICE, just in case I eliminated any of the chemotherapy drugs through my urine.

"This is important, Anita," the nurse said firmly. "We don't want to take a chance that anyone else might be exposed to the chemotherapy drugs."

The nurse accessed my port-a-cath, which hurt a little bit, but it wasn't that bad. I assumed the drugs would be dripped in from an IV bag, but instead she sat next to me and used a large syringe to "push" the drugs through the port.

The magnitude of chemotherapy is overwhelming. I get sick every time I think of it. Just writing this makes me nauseous. They put this poison into my body. Do you understand? They injected drugs that would melt the floor into my veins to destroy the rapidly-growing cells that were trying to kill me. But what else were they killing? My hair…yes…but what else? Seriously, no one can understand, really understand, unless you've been there. I can still smell the drugs. I can still taste them.

After the first round of chemotherapy, I felt relatively fine. I was a bit light-headed, but that's all. I thought this was going to be a breeze. All the horror stories were for other people, not me. I was told that twenty-four hours after each round of chemotherapy, I would need to return to the hospital for a shot of pegfilgrastim, a new drug sold under the trade name Neulasta. While Neulasta is frightfully expensive, it is an important designer drug used to boost white blood cells.

Chemotherapy works by killing off fast-growing cancer cells. There's one problem with this. Chemo drugs can't tell the difference between fast-growing cancer cells and fast-growing healthy ones. The healthy cells that may be killed off are your white and red blood cells. A low white blood cell count could lead to infection and a chance that I might not be able to get my next round of chemotherapy on time. I needed my blood counts to be "as close to normal" so that I could return for another round. Neulasta was the answer.

By the time I got home from my first shot of Neulasta, full body fatigue had set in and the first of a series of excruciatingly painful headaches began. *Oh, God, the horror stories are coming true.* For the next three days, my head stayed on the pillow; my bed was my best friend.

The first seventy-two hours after chemotherapy were the worst. It would be the world's greatest understatement to call those days "challenging." I quickly learned not to tough it out. I medicated the side effects as much as I could, especially the headaches. I have never had a migraine, but I can only assume that the pain is similar. I did not talk much. When I could stand the television being on, it was at a very low volume. Even my favorite old movies on TCM were too much to watch. *Cary Grant, Katharine Hepburn and Elizabeth Taylor will just have to wait.* I could not move too much or too fast. If we would have had a house fire on chemo weekends, I believe I would have been toast.

Thankfully, I was not stricken with nausea. Modern medicine is an awesome thing. "Just a couple of years ago," Dr. J told me, "a lot of patients would throw up almost immediately." I could see the sadness in his eyes as he continued. "In fact, I would send them into chemotherapy, and the nurses would have buckets ready for them." But thanks to the advent of anti-nausea drugs, I did not suffer that too.

Still, the irony of it all did not escape me: I was giving strangers permission to put poisons into my body in order to cure me. Oh, I was quite certain that I would be healed in the end. However, I did not fully comprehend that the "cure" would almost kill me.

There was one thing that I did not even think about when I was starting chemotherapy. I did not know I was to become one of the "sisterhood of survivors." It happened as my friends slowly learned of my diagnosis. One friend talked to another who talked to another and so on. Through this "chain," my phone number eventually was given to an absolutely incredible woman named Lorene Blohowiak.

There was a saying during the 1960s that was supposed to be the key to changing the world: *each one teach one.* If that is possible, then Lorene was my "teacher." Lorene is a survivor of metastatic breast cancer, and no one knows like another survivor. Lorene has fought the good fight and is still here, alive and kicking.

Lorene herself had been through hell, but that did not keep her from helping me. She had two small children and a husband at home, and she still found time to check on me after my chemotherapy treatments. She could sense when I needed to touch base with someone who "understood" my fears. My phone would ring, and we would talk for an hour. She was never in a rush, even though I know that her little kids needed tending to.

Lorene was, is, and always will be an inspiration to me. She sincerely cares about me and how I'm doing. Isn't it amazing how someone you did not know before diagnosis could have such a positive and powerful effect on you? How blessed I am to have her in my life.

The "sisterhood" also encompassed women who were not cancer survivors. Kim Schanock was another blessing in my life. I have known Kim since high school, for over 25 years. Before the advent of email, Kim and I would phone each other every six months and catch up on each other's lives. We would keep in touch, check out the latest personal and family news, send Christmas cards and letters, then go on with our similar but separate lives. Our friendship is the kind where you may not see each other for a long time, but when you do get together, you pick up as if no time had passed at all.

I believe Kim has always been on my path. She does, too. She tells me she had no idea why, but she was thinking of me in mid-August 2004, and decided to send a quick catch-up email. Her message reached me the first week I was diagnosed. I knew replying online was not the way to deliver the news, so I called her. We started with the same old, "Hey! How are you?" But this time, the conversation took a very different turn.

Kim took the news pretty hard because I am her friend and she loves me. There was that, of course, but there was also something else. As she said later, "The news was absolutely devastating because it's right there; someone you know, someone your own age has a life-threatening illness. If it could happen to Anita, it could happen to anyone. Even to me."

With all of those reasons factoring in, Kim committed herself to helping me in any way she could. She has been there for me every week since. I am not kidding. Whether it was food on chemotherapy weekends, a smiling voice on the other end of the phone, or help with household chores, her generosity is beyond words. I do not know what I did to deserve her, but I am so glad she is in my life.

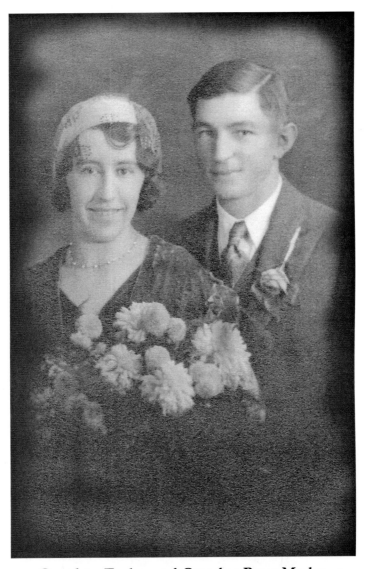

**Grandma Evelyn and Grandpa Peter Mathu
on their wedding day, October 26, 1932.
Grandma died October 5, 1954.
She was 45 years old.**

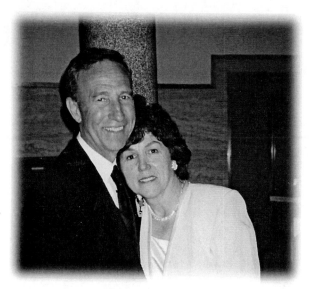

**Mom and Dad
April 2000**

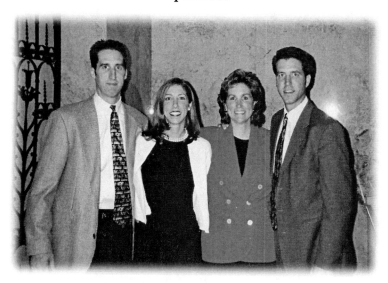

**The DuJardin Kids – April 2000
Matthew, Colleen, Anita and Jon**

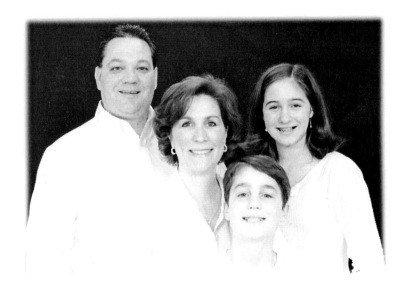

The Hockers
Ray, Anita, Tony, and Alyce

April 2004 ... 4 months before diagnosis

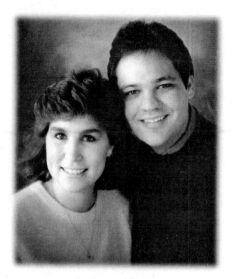

Anita and Ray
October 1986 Engagement

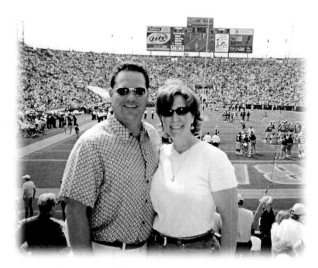

Ray and Anita
Green Bay Packers Game, Lambeau Field 2003

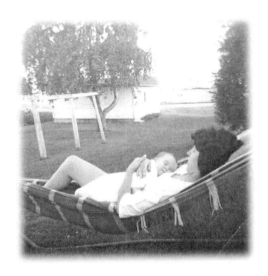

**Mom and Anita
July 1964**

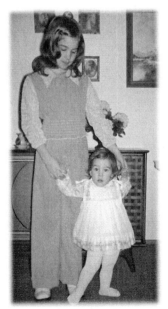

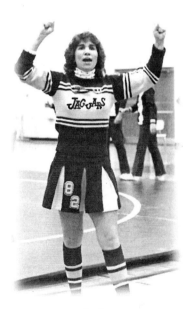

**Anita and Colleen
April 1974**

**Anita
1982**

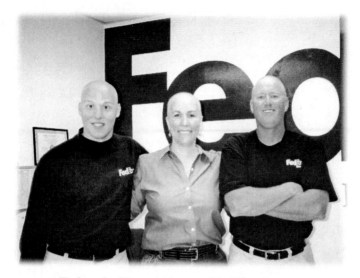

Being bald together at FedEx Ground
Andrew, Anita, and Jamie – September 2004

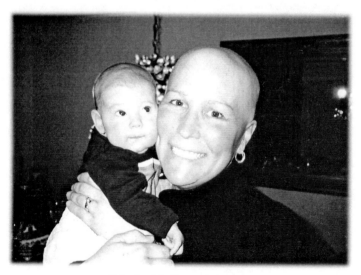

Little Neil and Anita
November 2004

Chapter 13

Just Like That, I Was Bald

When one door of happiness closes, another opens;
but often we look so long at the closed door that we do not see
the one which has been opened for us.
Helen Keller

The second round of chemotherapy happened to fall on the weekend of the Green Bay Packers home opener. I was crestfallen. Being a Packer fan in Green Bay is as natural as breathing. The DuJardins, like most Wisconsin families, are addicted to the Green and Gold. It starts in July when the preseason begins and doesn't end until the play-offs in January. It doesn't matter if the team wins or loses; the stadium is full, and Anita is there.

I never missed watching Brett Favre and the gang. Mom and Dad had been season ticket holders since the 1960s. When the Green Bay Packers opened up a children's section at Lambeau Field in the '70s, Dad was right there to sign his four children up for tickets. I believe that I was about ten years old when we received our season tickets, and I've been going to the games ever since. To show my utter devotion to the team, I attended a game when I was eight-and-a-half months pregnant with Alyce. Thanks to Alyce's arrival during a bye week, I did not miss a game. But this time, being at the home opener was not a possibility. I would have my chemotherapy on Thursday and would be glued to my bed on Sunday instead of cheering on the Packers at Lambeau.

So one of the "side effects" of my treatment was that my streak of never missing a Packer home game was to be broken. True, I was saved from seeing my beloved team suffer a humiliating defeat, but at the time, I was heartbroken to be missing the game. I didn't know I would soon experience another one of those *I-could-have-lived-without-this* moments. There were to be two devastating losses in Green Bay that weekend, and one would hit very close to home. The Packers lost at Lambeau, and Anita DuJardin Hockers would lose her hair.

Good thing I'm a low maintenance chick in the hair department. I'm not sure why, but my hair was never that big a deal to me, like it is for some women. Styling it was a part of my morning routine, and I liked the way it looked. I just didn't fuss with it that much. Hair was hair. Nonetheless, I was not prepared to encounter a "bad hair day" even my wildest imagination could not envision.

It was a sort of "Twilight Zone" moment. Cancer plays games with your mind. You want to think that all the side effects cannot happen to you, but most do. I was told that my hair would fall out fourteen days after my first round of chemotherapy. Right on schedule, fourteen days later, it did.

It was another Friday morning. I was in the shower, washing my hair, when my fingers got stuck. When I untangled them, strands and strands of hair came along. I just stood there dumbfounded, staring at this mass of hair in my hands. *My hair isn't supposed to fall out, all at once, on the same day!* I rinsed what was left on my head and got out of the shower. I called to Mom, who was downstairs, and said that it had begun. We exchanged one of those *you-have-got-to-be-kidding looks* and called Jane at the hair salon. Jane had been cutting my hair for years.

I tried to be cool, but I know my voice must have been frantic. "Jane, this is Anita Hockers. Do you have anything open this afternoon?"

"Let me check, Anita."

"Please Jane. Try to squeeze me in. I didn't want to tell you this way, but I have breast cancer. I'm on chemo, and my hair started falling out this morning. I don't know what to do."

Silence. It's so difficult telling people over the phone that you have cancer. Inevitably, there's an awkward silence on the other end of the line. Then reality sets in and you finish the conversation.

"Of course," she finally said. "Can you be here by two-thirty?"

Jane was patient with me. I was mad, really mad. I couldn't believe I had to shave my head, but I decided right then and there to get it over with. "I want it off," I said. "Now. No screwing around; take it all off."

The alternative was to have my hair fall out daily, to be shocked every time I looked in the mirror. A lot of cancer patients decide to go this route, but I just could not do it. Jane, bless her heart, did what I asked. And just like that, I was bald.

Once my hair was gone, it wasn't as bad as I thought it would be. I had always said, "If I ever have cancer, I will not wear a wig." And I didn't. As a matter of fact, everyone I met told me I looked pretty good bald. It may sound like bragging, but I have to say I agreed. People marveled at the roundness of my head, which has no dents or divots. My 83-year-old neighbor, Fern, said, "Well Anita, look at that head. Your mom must have turned you a lot when you were a baby." Mom and I giggled when I told her what Fern had said. That must have been it!

Holly Weiske came over that night. Holly is one of my dearest friends. She has seen me at my best and at my worst. I had nearly convinced myself that I did look pretty good bald, but seeing the reaction in my girlfriend's eyes would tell me the truth. Holly walked in and smiled. She said, "This has got to be a joke, woman. You look better than I do during a good-hair day! You rock, sister-friend." Those were the words I needed to hear. Even my heart smiled.

I have heard from many of my nurses that I was brave to walk around with my bald head. No wig, no hat. My nurse Connie said that many women simply cannot do it. They need to wear a wig for themselves, to boost their self-esteem as they battle this disease. They need to seem normal to the outside world. But on the flip side, I bet that some women wear wigs, not for themselves, but for other people. It puts other people at ease; the people they encounter do not have to confront their own fears about cancer and chemotherapy by looking at a bald female. For me, none of that mattered. My bald head was my badge of courage, and I was going to wear it with pride. I was determined not to let being bald stop me.

As I said, being bald is not so bad. It certainly was nothing compared to what happened to my body that Sunday after my second round of chemotherapy. Pre-cancer, I would have been at the Packer game, very happy and very hydrated. But instead, here I was, down flat in bed, bald, unable and unwilling to move. I admit it was my own fault. I fell prey to the dreaded "dehydration."

Dr. J and the nurses had told me more than once to get plenty of fluids, but lying in bed, I forgot. Actually, I was so tired and in so much pain, I wanted only to lie there, to do nothing but stay in my bed. It took too much effort to sit up, even to take those essential sips of juice or water. Very foolishly, I didn't force myself. Suddenly, my body got very warm, and I was perspiring profusely. Then my heart began to race. I was sure I was having a heart attack. Moments later, Ray and I were headed to the ER.

A bald, cancer patient in such an obviously critical state commands special attention in a hospital emergency room. No waiting for me. I like attention; who doesn't? It was my time to get a lot of it. I was dehydrated and probably in a bit of danger, but a simple procedure saved me from feeling any worse. The nurses hooked up the heart monitor and started an IV drip. The liquid flowed slowly into my veins, bringing my fluid levels back to normal and restoring my metabolic functions. Too bad something similar wasn't happening across town. It was Sunday, and every television in the place was tuned to the same channel. I had to sit there, attached to a machine, and watch in disgust as the Chicago Bears beat the Packers at Lambeau. It would be blatantly redundant to mention it, but I can't resist. We were both having a very bad day.

Poor jokes aside, my third and fourth rounds of adriamycin and cytoxan entailed more of the same, except that it got progressively worse. There is no getting around it. The cumulative effects of chemotherapy are exhausting. Somehow I dealt with the fatigue, but I was plagued by horrible bouts of constipation. My world consisted of my bedroom and my bathroom. I moved back and forth, going nowhere else during chemo weekends. I did not venture downstairs. I stayed where I was most comfortable and protected, in my bed. It took all my strength to talk to my children. Ray and the kids brought me kisses and glasses of water; that was all I needed at the time.

Chapter 14

Bald, Bumpy and Beautiful

The smallest of kindnesses can be the greatest of gifts.
Anonymous

Wisconsin was steeling itself for another bout with old man Winter, and the Packers were enjoying another winning season as I was getting ready for my fifth round of chemotherapy. As usual though, I had to see Dr. J first. During each exam before chemotherapy, he would palpate my breast, trying to assess whether or not there were any changes in the tumors. Every time I went to his office, I anxiously awaited his signature expression, "Good, good, good. This is good." That remark indicated that he was very happy with my progress; the tumors seemed to be shrinking.

That particular day, I was not my usual self. I felt down and defeated, worn out and depressed from the toll the chemicals had taken on my body. It was a surprising lapse for someone so positive, but I did have an occasional bout of well-deserved self-pity. Anyway, as Dr. J began the customary examination of my right breast, I felt emotionally and physically drained. What a difference a few moments can make! My spirits lifted immediately when he looked at me and smiled, "Good, good, good. You're ready for your fifth round, Anita. You're responding excellently to chemotherapy."

Suddenly, I was on top of the world! All my suffering was paying off. Everything was going as planned. I left his office more determined than ever to see this thing through. *I will do whatever it takes. I will survive.* Little did I know that the *worst* was not behind me. I had no idea how much more agony the *"whatever it takes"* would entail.

I began my series of Taxotere two weeks after the fourth round of adriamycin and cytoxan. This regimen started exactly like the first drugs, but with Taxotere, I was on a once-every-three-weeks schedule. Taxotere is extremely toxic, which is why it can only be administered every twenty-one days. It also has some strange side effects. "That drug's going to knock you on your ass and take your fingernails too," another chemo patient told me with ominous, knowing eyes. I prayed that those side effects wouldn't happen to me. The hair was enough, right? Wrong.

Each chemotherapy drug is administered a bit differently. Though I had adriamycin and cytoxan pushed into me through my port using a large syringe, Taxotere was dripped in with an IV bag. First the anti-nausea drug, wait twenty minutes, then the Taxotere. I felt a bit weak and light-headed during the treatment, but I kept telling myself that I was over halfway there. Five down, three to go.

Just a few hours after the first dose, I knew that chemo patient had been right. I lay in bed, totally unable to believe what was happening to my body. My hands and feet hurt in a way I never thought possible. My hands throbbed. I tried to lie on my back with my arms right next to my body. I figured that if they were in that position, the pain would go away. I was wrong. It was excruciating. My hands hurt so much I couldn't stand it. But that wasn't all. My feet were also tender to the touch; it hurt to even move them. Just having a lightweight sheet covering them felt like a twenty-pound weight was pressing down upon them.

I tried all kinds of non-medicinal things to ease the pain. Warm bath, hot shower, but nothing helped. Finally, in desperation, I self-medicated with pain pills. That gave me some blessed relief, and I was able to sleep a little here and there.

When I had to leave my bed, walking was very difficult. I hurt all over; I was exhausted and terribly weak. I hated to ask, but Ray had to help me go to the bathroom. *Nice, real nice. I'm forty years old and need help going potty!* I felt so helpless, but I was determined to try to continue on with my life. Fortunately, every day the side effects lessened, and I began to feel better.

Being the trooper that I am, I got up to go to work four days after my first round of Taxotere. I had gone to work within a few days of my previous chemo treatments, and I did not even consider staying home this time. Driving to work I thought, *"I'm so weak; I really shouldn't be on the road."* I swear it was almost like drunk driving. How stupid of me to risk my life and the lives of others in an attempt to be some kind of gotta-go-to-work hero.

As soon as I arrived and sat down at my desk, the boys at FedEx Ground knew something was wrong. I put my head on the desk and carefully placed my hands on my lap because the pain was unbearable. My hands were showing the classic side effects of Taxotere; they were literally burning from the inside out. The boys moved quickly, and twenty minutes later I was at the hospital. They had called Ray, and he was waiting for me when I walked in. We both went in to see Dr. J. He looked right at me, like he always does, and I knew he truly felt for me. He knows this treatment is terrible and makes no excuses for it.

"Anita, remember when I told you this cancer will change your life forever?" he asked with gentle, empathetic eyes. "That you will never be the same or look at things the same again?" I nodded, unable to hold back my tears. "You have got to stop trying to be so brave."

"It's just that I want my life back, that I…" The rest was lost in my sobs. He let me weep until I regained my composure enough to mumble, "I'm sorry for crying like this. I feel like such a baby…"

He took my hand and said, "Stop. You don't have to apologize for crying, to me or anyone else. Crying is good. You have things to cry about." What a sweet man. He knew just what I needed to hear.

Dr. J's words reminded me of Sherrie's dad who had also said things I needed to hear. Sherrie Schoen, my partner in crime, my high school cheerleading pal, one of my dearest and oldest friends. Sherrie was having her own challenges while I was going through chemotherapy. About the time I was diagnosed, Sherrie's father had just come out of remission. He was very ill, but when Sherrie told him about me, he found the strength to call me and ask how I was doing. This man was very sick, and still he called me.

That conversation is something I will always remember. Mr. Smits was a man of such faith; he never once doubted God. "Anita, I never thought that I was going to end up in this predicament," he told me in a weak voice that was just above a whisper. "I should be out there cutting my grass, playing with my dog, and watching my grandchildren grow up. But I'm here, and maybe it's my job to tell you that everything is going to be all right. God has a plan; we are not suffering in vain."

"Maybe God has a plan, Mr. Smits, but dammit, why is all this suffering necessary to find out what it is?"

I could feel him smile through the phone. "There is a plan, Anita. I guarantee it. Trust God." He died four weeks after that phone call. Sherrie's sadness enveloped her, but she was still there for me. Using her Dad's strength, she made me laugh on many a dreary day. Sherrie is the poster child for devoted friendship. If only her Dad was here so I could tell him how much his words and his daughter mean to me. But then I think he knows.

Within a week, my hands lost their first layer of skin. The skin came off in sheets. It's hard to describe, all I can say is that somehow I lived through the horror of watching my body slowly disintegrate, often discarding parts that fell off into the waste basket as if they were useless garbage.

Taxotere number two and three were the same; I was completely exhausted. Now the effects of all the chemotherapy really began to show. My bald head was still cute, but the rest was not so attractive. My eyebrows were very thin and my eyelashes fell out completely. I had been prescribed some steroids to combat some of the side effects of Taxotere. The medication made my face break out in big, hard bumps. These were not pimples. They were large bumps. I was bald, weak, and mentally challenged. I did not need hideous-looking bumps on my face, too.

Then something happened that I will never forget. It was in November, between my sixth and seventh rounds of chemo. I was actually starting to get used to my ghastly appearance. Feeling and looking like death warmed over was becoming the norm. The guys at FedEx Ground must have been put off by my appearance, but they never skipped a beat. They still told me their stupid jokes and tried to make me laugh as much as possible. They were and continue to be simply the best.

During one of my tougher days, my boss Kevin walked out of his office and asked innocently, "What're you doing tomorrow, Anita?"

"Getting my hair done; having a facial," I said with a smart-ass grin, trying to be the "old" Anita.

"Too bad. Favre's been named FedEx Ground Player of the Week." Brett had been phenomenal in the Green Bay win over the Minnesota Vikings. "I'm presenting him with the award and a check tomorrow and was wondering if you'd like to go along and meet him."

Finally it was some GOOD fortune that had come my way. "You have got to be kidding! Meet Brett Favre? Of course I'll go…I'd be honored!" *Me? Meet Brett Favre? I just might faint!*

The next day Kevin and I walked into the media conference room at Lambeau Field where Brett was preparing for his weekly Wednesday press conference. The plan was that we would present the award before the Q and A session. Brett would accept the money in honor of his charity, the Brett Favre Fourward Foundation.

Honestly, I was a little more than nervous for two reasons. One, this was Brett Favre, for heaven's sake; and two, I didn't know how Brett would react to my appearance. I knew his wife Deanna had just made public the news that she would be fighting her own battle with breast cancer. And there I would be—bald, bumpy, beautiful Anita.

Right on time, Brett came out to meet us. He was dressed in his usual baseball cap, T-shirt, and shorts. He looked me right in the eye and shook my hand. I congratulated him on a good game, and we handed him his check. Imagine that. His wife was beginning chemotherapy that week, and standing here in front of him was a bald chick who was obviously a cancer patient. Yet he was very gracious and never missed a beat.

It's weird, but I thought when I actually met the man a lot of people in Green Bay consider the greatest Green Bay Packer EVER, I would be awe-struck. But I wasn't. Famous people, especially athletes, always seem bigger than life. But he wasn't. My brothers are both over 6 feet tall, and Brett did not look much bigger. *He's just a guy. A guy who can throw a great spiral. A guy who can take Green Bay fans to their knees on any given Sunday. A sure-bet for the Hall of Fame. And a guy whose wife has breast cancer. Sure does level the playing field, doesn't it?*

I really wanted my picture taken with him. I had talked to the staff photographer before Brett arrived and politely asked if he thought Brett would mind having his picture taken with a bald lady. He smiled and thought that Brett would oblige. But it didn't happen. Brett's press conference was about to begin, and he had very little time for pleasantries. He walked away before I could even ask him. I watched as he approached the podium, adjusted his cap, talked about the game, and took questions from the reporters.

Kevin had told me Brett always wrapped up his press conferences quickly. If there were no more questions, he would exit, stage left, in a flash. This day ran true to form. He was almost through the door when I called his name. He turned around and walked back toward me. I asked him if he would mind having his picture taken with me. He smiled and said, "Sure." That one little word brightened my spirit in a way Brett will never know.

It only took a minute. We posed quickly, and the staff photographer snapped away. I will always cherish that photo and that "Kodak moment." Brett's small gesture of kindness spread sunshine in my life that lasted until Christmas. After all, how many chicks, bald or otherwise, get their picture taken with "the man" in Green Bay?

Speaking of Christmas, the holiday season of 2004 was not the customary bright lights, glittering parties, power shopping, and oodles of presents under the tree for me. I had finished my seventh round of chemotherapy and was gearing up for the last one. Per family tradition, Anita, Jon, Matt, and Colleen arrived at my parents' house on Christmas Day with our families in tow. We love our family Christmases together, but for the first time in my life, I could not get in the holiday mood. I wanted so badly to relax and enjoy the day, but I felt horrible. I managed somehow to put on my "happy" face. I recall thinking, *"Everyone looks like a million bucks today, but I feel and look like shit!"* Still, I needed to show them all that I would just "get this done," that I would "kick this cancer-thing."

After all, I did not want anyone worrying. I wanted to have the kind of Christmas we always had: laughs, drinks, and good times. Behind their smiles, I know that they were all concerned. *Maybe if we don't talk about it, it won't be real.* But the worry cloud was there, everyone could feel it.

I tried my best to be strong. But you know what? I wasn't that strong. I looked like hell, I was weaker than I had ever been in my life, and I was scared, too. I was facing the likely prospect that if the chemotherapy cocktail had done its job of shrinking the tumors, my good fortune meant that in just three weeks a surgeon would remove a significant portion of my body.

Somehow I stumbled through that Christmas season. I was going to celebrate the arrival of the New Year with no idea what 2005 would bring, though I was very happy that 2004 was gone forever.

When my final round of chemotherapy came the day before New Year's Eve, I marked it with another milestone. As I sat in the clinic, awaiting my treatment, I lost my first fingernail. My nails didn't fall off, but rather peeled off, from right to left. It's hard to accurately describe how they looked, but by the time they fell off, each of my fingernails had four ridges on them. It seemed to me that the nail would be shocked with each round of Taxotere, sink in, and die a little; then try to heal itself during the next three weeks. It occurred to me that my fingernails were behaving just like I felt. I would endure a round of chemotherapy, sink in, die a little, and then try to heal before the next one.

But all good (and bad) things come to an end. It was finally over. I went home to bed that day and tried to get my arms around the fact that surgery was just around the corner, that my body was about to be changed forever.

Chapter 15

Gonna Take a Bullet

If you light a lamp for somebody, it will also brighten your path.
Buddhist Proverb

I believe it may be harder to be the loved one of someone who is sick than it is to be the person who is ill. I really do. I know it was rough on my loved ones, especially my children. It didn't take Alyce and Tony long to guess there was something seriously wrong on that fateful August day. I remember finally going into the house and standing in the doorway of the den, my face red and swollen from crying. For a moment, I just looked at them both. Then it took all my strength to say, "Kids. Bad news. I have cancer."

I could almost feel the air being sucked out of the room. They had tears in their eyes, but they didn't panic. It was hard, but I said with as much conviction as I could muster, "I have cancer, but I am not going anywhere. Do you hear me? I am not going anywhere. It won't be easy, but I will beat this."

It won't be easy. No shit. It was hard for my children to see me sick. It was hard for me to put a smile on everyday, to let them know I would be all right. It was hard for them to have a bald mom.

Alyce was barely fourteen. It's difficult enough being a teenager these days, much less dealing with a mother who has breast cancer. But like me, Alyce is a strong young woman. She's also as smart as they come, with a wonderful personality. She made sure that, if I was well enough, I was present at every school function, bald head and all. She loves me and was proud of me, battling this disease, and I am so proud of her.

Tony was only ten when I was diagnosed, and he was very scared. Tony is my baby. He's my "little man of very few words," and he loves his mom with all his heart. I could read his mind from the look on his face. This was not supposed to be happening to his mom! His eyes welled up with tears, but all he could do, and all that he needed to do, was to hug me.

Tony didn't react to my baldness the same way Alyce did. One day when I picked him up from school, he gave me a strange look and asked, "Mom, can you wear a hat when you pick me up?" I thought that was pretty powerful. I don't really think he was embarrassed by my appearance. In fact, I think he was trying to *protect* me because he thought I might be embarrassed if one of the kids made a comment. My kids must have inherited their strength from me. I know that they got their huge, loving hearts from Ray.

Ray. How does a spouse really feel when his or her "other half" is so ill? You'll never know unless you're put in that situation. It may not be true everywhere, but in our Midwestern Green Bay setting, husbands still have the traditional role in the family. The man of the house is supposed to have Herculean strength that can shoulder any burden. He's got to provide for his wife and kids; put a roof over their heads and food on the table; make excellent decisions, fix things when they break; in other words, be a **man** in every sense of the word.

Ray never missed a cue before my diagnosis, but now he needed to add to his list all the housework and errands that I was accustomed to doing. He worked, picked up the kids, cooked, cleaned, did the laundry, and still made me feel special. I know he thought he had to do it all when I got sick, but it was not physically possible. For instance, it upset him that he couldn't be at all the appointments, all the treatments. But there weren't enough hours in the day. "Besides," I told him more than once, "I need you more *after* the appointments."

It was hard at first for Ray to accept assistance from other people. We have always been a fiercely independent, self-sufficient couple. When Jane Kozicki called to inform us that a "meal brigade" had been set up during chemotherapy weekends, we were overwhelmed. Jane knew all too well what the power of food could do. Her sister-in-law had fought this breast cancer monster two years ago. Jane had set up the same meal brigade for her and knew that Ray, even though he protested, would need her assistance. Ray said he was appreciative of her kind gesture, but leaned toward politely refusing the extra help. Actually, we felt guilty. However, when we sat down and really thought about it, we realized that we couldn't do this alone. After that, we gratefully accepted whatever people wanted to do for us. They needed to help, and we needed to let them. It was the right thing to do.

Speaking of doing the right thing. Following Jane's meal brigade deliveries, the girls on my volleyball team instituted "meals on wheels" during my recovery from surgery. It couldn't have come at a better time. Their first delivery came on a day when Ray had come home from picking up the kids, grocery shopping, and stopping at the pharmacy for my pain medication. I was in bed, and the doorbell rang. Mary Koehler was there with a ready-to-reheat-and-eat meal. What a relief! As she pulled dish after dish of delicious-looking food out of her cooler, Ray couldn't resist…he hugged her. To tell the honest to God's truth, I think I saw tears of gratitude in his eyes.

Right before she left, Mary embraced me fiercely and looked me straight in the eye. "You are not going anywhere, Anita," she said emphatically. "It's gonna take a bullet to get rid of you." *Now that's the truth. And might I add, a well-placed bullet to boot.*

Bringing meals gave our friends a chance to feel they were doing something for us. Let me tell you, I don't think my family has eaten better food before or since. Most of the time, people don't know what to say or do during an illness. But really, it doesn't take much to tell us that you care. A phone call, a card, flowers, or food will brighten a down day for someone who is fighting for her life. When misfortune strikes a relative, friend, or neighbor, and you feel that there is nothing you can say or do, do something. I will say it once again: doing anything is the right thing to do.

The extraordinary kindness of our friends made us realize one more thing. Maybe *we* had made a difference in their lives, too. Maybe they went home and appreciated their family and friends just a little bit more. If there is a higher purpose for my illness, I surely hope it is the realization that this can happen to anyone.

You might recall that I said in the beginning of this book that the DuJardins—my family—have always been very close. We have always hugged, kissed, and basically smothered each other. So it comes as no surprise that, after the initial shock of learning I had cancer, they got down to business, helping out in whatever way they could.

Without being asked, Dad and Mom came over and pitched in. They also "stormed heaven" with prayers for my complete recovery. Dad took to calling me every day just to see if I needed anything. Mom was at every appointment and chemotherapy treatment except one. Mom wanted to be there that day, and I felt her presence. She was there in spirit, if not in person. Dad told me she tried, but she could not get up off the couch. She was recuperating from major surgery ordered after the genetic testing: a preventative hysterectomy designed to keep her from having cancer. It was bad enough that her beloved oldest daughter had it. She would prevent it from happening to her any way she could.

Colleen was in Green Bay that first week to meet with my trio of doctors, but she had to go back to Chicago after the consultations. I cannot imagine how hard it must have been to leave someone you love who is hurting. But her life was still out there. She could not put her job, her life, on hold. She returned to Green Bay after the first round of chemotherapy. She was there when the headaches started on that first, dreadful Saturday. She put her head on the pillow next to me and cried. She called me every day, and made sure I had fresh flowers and cards to fill those crazy chemotherapy weekends.

I know that she secretly wished I would wear a wig, maybe a long blonde one. She probably would have preferred that I put make-up on my face even though I did not have eyelashes. But she never once second-guessed my decisions. She followed my wishes, smiled at my bald head, and marveled at my strength. She will always be my little angel.

It goes without saying that my brothers, Jon and Matt, were very worried about me, too. Jon is a year younger than I am; he's the tough guy. He puts on a brave face, but I know my illness affected him. Proof positive is the phone call I got when he had a son while I was going through chemotherapy. I felt so bad that I couldn't be there when the baby was born. I'm the sister who is always on top of everything. I am always there when something happens in our family.

However, during this time, I and everyone else had to be content with good wishes expressed through phone calls. On that unforgettable day when Jon called to tell me Little Neil had arrived, we cried together. But this time the tears were shed in happiness. It was so good to have something positive happening in the DuJardin family. Neil's birth proved once again that this world keeps spinning, no matter how badly we want it to stop.

Another very important person in my support system is my little brother Matt. Matt is four years younger and has always been a softie, such a puddle. He's a sweet, wonderful man, there whenever I need him. When I called to tell him I had cancer, his voice broke. "Okay, let's just get one thing straight right away, Anita," he said. I know there were tears in his eyes. "I need my big sister. I will be there for you, always." And he has. He has driven three hours just to say hello and rub my bald head. Jon and Matt are my brothers and they are my friends. Thinking back to that day at Grandma's house, I am glad that my "dirty looks" didn't do any harm.

Speaking of brothers. Though "the boys" at FedEx Ground are not blood relatives, they belong in my extraordinary support group, and I cannot finish this chapter without mentioning them. I call them "the boys" because they are indeed like brothers to me.

Two days after I was diagnosed, when I told my boss, I was very nervous. I did **not** want to cry. I closed the door of his office and nervously said, "I have cancer." Kevin didn't even flinch. His demeanor did not change one bit when I explained about my illness. He smiled and made it known from that day forward, I would not have to worry about my job. I need only worry about getting better.

I tried hard to return his loyalty. Except for each Friday after my Thursday chemotherapy sessions, I worked every single day. Kevin continually kept a protective eye on me. He was the first one to tell me to go home when I looked like I couldn't function anymore. He never questioned me. He's much more than my boss; he's my friend.

The rest of the guys at work were equally supportive. The day I walked into the office with a bald head, the boys grinned and said that I looked great. I am smiling just thinking about this. The very next day those men showed me the power of teamwork. When I walked into work the next morning, I was not the only bald person at FedEx Ground. We were all bald. I will never be able to repay them for the support and kindness they showed me during those long months.

Chapter 16

One Step Away From Being a Dude

*Hope is the golden thread that should be woven
into every experience of life.*
Unknown

Surgery was scheduled for January 18, 2005. I knew about the date for a couple of weeks but did not tell anyone except my family and closest friends. I don't know why. I just didn't want to talk about it. All I had been doing was talking about cancer, about being bald, about losing my hair, about losing my boobs. I was just so tired, so sick of it all. Sick and tired of being sick and tired.

I had an appointment with Dr. Colette the day before surgery. She walked me through the procedure and asked if I had any questions or concerns. Impulsively, I asked her something that had been on my mind since August. "Were these tumors missed on the mammogram I had last June?"

"Well, let's go across the hall and look at the films. They're digital so we'll have no problem finding your views."

She motioned to me to follow her. As Ray and Mom trudged along, I watched them exchange glances that said *I cannot believe she just asked that question!*

Once we accessed the file, the views popped up on the computer immediately. They were mine; in the right-hand corner was typed, *Hockers, Anita M., 40-year-old, Female.* Dr. Colette scanned them and pulled up the other views they had taken that day. She spent some time looking at them. She did not say what I expected to hear, *"Yes, they were right. No tumors detected."*

Instead she said, "Well, Anita, I'm not kidding you, but I think you could have driven a bus behind your boobs and we would not have been able to see it." I gave her a quizzical look and then started to laugh. Ray smiled, and Mom laughed just as hard as I did.

She went on. "Because your breasts were fibro-cystic and so dense, they read the films correctly. If the tumors were there in June, they were not visible on your mammogram." Dr. Colette waited for my response. I was so relieved that I just nodded my head, at last secure in the knowledge that there had been no human error involved in not finding my cancer sooner. *Okay, I can finally put those fears to rest. Besides, I have much bigger things to be concerned about for tomorrow.*

The surgery would be performed in two parts: first a complete hysterectomy and then a bilateral mastectomy. Hormones, especially estrogen, play a key role in the development and spread of cancer. The idea was to remove every part of me that might produce estrogen, thus causing the cancer to recur. *Sweet. Just one step away from being a dude…*

I blithely walked into the hospital as if it was any other cold day in snow-covered Northeastern Wisconsin. One would have thought that I was going for a manicure or pedicure, anything besides major surgery. I remember that day like it was yesterday. I cannot imagine why I was not scared out of my mind as I got undressed. I wonder now why I was not kicking and screaming that day. Instead, I went in there so calmly. I stripped down, put on a gown, peed in a cup, and let them do their thing.

Maybe I was getting used to being out of control, letting others handle the situation. Does the brain shut off during times like these? Shut off and let it all happen? *I just have to trust my doctors and the powers that be. I have with me the people who mean the most to me; what else is there to worry about?*

As usual, I started joking with the staff, about not being able to pee, about how my gown was going to fit much better after surgery, about wanting drugs right now! Okay, that wasn't a joke. All of a sudden, it hit me. I considered the full impact of what was about to happen, and I knew. I was joking around because I was scared to death.

Dr. Mike handled the first phase, a laparoscopic assisted vaginal hysterectomy with bilateral salpingo-oophorectomy. All this means is that he removed my uterus, ovaries, and fallopian tubes. He made three incisions in my belly for the scope to assist him. Removing these parts does sound a bit barbaric, but risking the alternative, another bout with cancer, was not an option.

When Dr. Mike finished his portion of the surgery, he handed me off to Dr. Colette. I lost a lot of blood during the first phase of the operation, which made things a bit dicey for a while. In fact, Dr. Colette was not sure she should proceed with the mastectomies. She told me later that she had consulted with Dr. Mike before deciding to continue on with the second phase: a bilateral mastectomy.

When my Grandma Evelyn had her surgery, the most common surgery was the radical mastectomy. It involved removal of the breast, all surrounding lymph nodes up to the collarbone, and the underlying chest muscle. This surgery is rarely performed today. It was developed in the late 1800s, when it was thought that more extensive surgery would most likely stop the cancer.

It goes without saying that Grandma Evelyn was left highly disfigured by her radical mastectomy. Many women were left with a large depression in their chest wall from this operation, which at times would require skin grafting to cover. This type of surgery was also known to significantly decrease arm sensation and motion.

Thank heavens I had the contemporary surgery of choice: modified radical mastectomy. The surgeon removes breast tissue, the nipple, an ellipse of skin, and some or all of the axillary or underarm lymph nodes, but leaves the chest muscle intact. I was told that this method would leave me with a more normal chest. Dr. Colette knew that I was not reconstructing and that I would want the flattest chest possible.

There are many, many women who are able to have a lumpectomy. I was not one of them. Dr. Colette explained that a lumpectomy was not an option because I had three tumors in two different quadrants of the right breast. Therefore, the entire breast had to be removed. "You will be too disfigured if I remove only half your breast," she explained, "and besides, it's really your best insurance against recurrence to have ALL the breast tissue removed."

It may seem extreme, but as a precautionary move, I elected to have my left breast removed at the same time. There was no sign of cancer there, but I chose this route for purely preventative reasons. If I had not, the chance of me having cancer in the left breast was just too much for me to risk.

The removal of my breasts went off without a hitch. I was in surgery the entire day, under anesthesia for almost seven hours. It's hard to believe that you can be put to sleep for that long and come out of it alive. However, when I did awaken, I felt like a Mack truck had hit me. I remember very little of that day, but I do recall Mom, Dad, Colleen, Aunt Colette, Ray, and little brother Matt being there in the recovery room. What I will never forget is the look of fear on their faces. They tell me that I was blue-gray and lifeless. Aunt Colette told me later that I looked very still and very flat. Imagine that. I have always had big boobs and now my chest was flat…flat as the gurney I was lying upon. Colleen said she gets chills thinking about how terrible I looked. Mom tries not to think about it. Ray smiles. I was alive. Ray always smiles when he thinks of that.

During my first night of recovery, Dr. Colette called my room. The nurses had informed her that my blood count was dangerously low. I was so weak I could hardly hold the phone to talk to her. As I listened, her voice sounded grim. "Anita, I think you should be given some blood," she said. "It may take weeks for your body to replace what you lost during the hysterectomy."

I mumbled something like, "You want me to put somebody else's blood into my body?"

She seemed unfazed by my concern, more worried about what might happen if I didn't. "I'm concerned about infection, maybe other potential complications if you don't." She knew how mind and body-bending the surgery was and did not want me fighting anything else.

"But…" I was not crazy about the idea because I had heard horror stories about tainted blood being given during transfusions. I didn't appreciate the idea that hepatitis or AIDS cells might replace the cancerous ones I had battled for months.

"It's safe. Really. Loss of blood can be easily fixed," she reassured me. "And it is safe, Anita. That's what blood banks are for. Two pints should do the trick." Then she added, "It's up to you, Anita, but if you don't, your recovery could be much harder and longer."

Doesn't everyone wince at the thought of someone else's blood flowing through his or her veins? But the facts were right in front of me…I needed it. I was convinced and did as Dr. Colette recommended.

Lying there that night, I watched in amazement as two nurses administered the blood. This transfusion process is obviously serious business. The nurses checked, double-checked, and triple-checked my hospital wristband against the paperwork. Then they triple-checked the numbers on the bags of blood. One nurse read them, the other wrote them down. Then they switched paperwork and repeated the process.

There was not one tiny step of protocol missed before, during, or after they hooked me up to receive the blood.

I felt a little stronger the next day, but I had a very hard time breathing. Seven hours of surgery will do a number on the healthy organs in your body. Dr. Colette told me my diaphragm "went to sleep" during surgery and did not push my lungs as it normally would. The result was common and predictable: my lungs had partially collapsed during the long surgery. This meant I had to exercise to get my lungs working again. It wasn't easy. It hurt to breathe. My mastectomies really didn't hurt, and neither did my lower half, but man, did it hurt to breathe.

It was pure torture, but I did the breathing exercises they recommended to get things back to normal again. I had to blow into a little contraption, using my breath to push a small ball up to the top. I blew as hard as I could. Nothing. I tried again. It moved a tiny fraction of an inch. Once more. I managed to move the ball up by about an inch. It hurt to laugh but Colleen and I giggled. "Guess we have some work to do," she joked.

Sometime that day, Dr. Colette called with the pathology report. I took a deep breath, winced from the discomfort, and braced myself. Mom and Colleen were sitting next to me as Dr. Colette read the report to me over the phone. Neoadjuvant chemotherapy had done its job. According to the pathologist, there was no sign of cancer in the breasts or the tissues that had been removed. He could see where the tumor sites had been, but tests done during surgery did not detect any remaining malignant cells. *Margins: negative for malignancy. 19 lymph nodes: negative for malignancy. Skin and adipose tissue: negative for malignancy.* That meant I was in remission. That was a good phone call. No. That was a GREAT phone call.

On the third day, I got my lungs back. The breathing exercises had done the deed; I was able to breathe freely and without discomfort. Now I could concentrate on my other parts, my missing parts. As I said before, I had lived with large breasts for almost three decades. (I later found out that they weighed about three pounds each. Yes, try putting six one-pound packages of hamburger meat on your chest and walk around all day, every day, like that). Now I had a new body to deal with.

It wasn't as if I was mourning the loss of my breasts, but by the middle of that third day, I hadn't looked at my chest yet because I was too scared. Who wouldn't be? Of course I thought about looking. In fact, at times that was the only thing on my mind. But I had no idea what to expect and I didn't have the courage. I would start to peek down my shirt, but then I'd say to myself, "No, not right now. I'm not ready." I chastised myself. *Some tough-chick you are, Anita! You can't even look at your own body!*

Unfortunately and inaccurately, when I pictured what I might look like, it was Grandma Evelyn or other women who had undergone radical mastectomies that I envisioned. That's probably the main reason I hadn't sought out any pictures of survivors. I did not want to see their scars. It might have been my subconscious that willfully left me in the dark without a clue as to what my front side would look like. Yes, I wanted to be left in the dark on this one.

Then, too, no cancer survivor had ever offered to show me her mastectomy scars. Really, it's not the kind of request you make of someone who has had this operation. Plus, I had never asked my doctors to give me a glimpse of a typical post-operative chest. I suppose it was like being an ostrich with her head in the sand, but at the time I figured que sera, sera. What will be will be. *I have chemotherapy to deal with. That's bad enough.*

Dr. Colette put an end to the whole issue on the afternoon of the third day when she came in to check on me. "Let's take a look," she said with a big smile on her face. We opened up my shirt, and I was pleasantly surprised. There was one long massive scar from armpit to armpit, with about a two-inch space in the middle. My chest was not concave! I was thrilled about that because having boobs that stick out is one thing. Being flat-chested is one thing. Living with a depression where your boobs are supposed to be is quite another.

All in all, it wasn't that bad. The only thing that made me uncomfortable was the presence of four separate drains that were hanging out of the sides of my chest. They were to stay in until the fluid from my chest stopped draining. Dr. Colette said it would take about two weeks. She also cautioned that it would take months, even years for the healing process to be complete. I would have numbness and would need therapy to loosen the tightness in my chest muscles, but I would recover. I felt the tears rise as I thanked God for those wonderful words. I didn't care if my boobs were gone. I never wanted to pose for *Playboy Magazine* anyway. I just wanted to live.

Colleen had to go home to Chicago that night. Saying goodbye to her was heartbreaking. Sigh. She had managed to put her fears of needles and medical treatments aside. If you haven't been poked and prodded like I've been, there is a fear of the unknown. Colleen sat next to me all day at the hospital and made me smile through the pain. She and Mom watched my every move, even when I had to use the toilet. They grabbed my IV pole and helped me shuffle to the bathroom. There's absolutely no modesty to contend with after what I had just gone through. I am sure they felt as helpless as I did, but they never showed it. Thinking back to those days in the hospital makes me realize, once again, how glad I am that I had my Mom with me. I was also eternally grateful that she and Dad had given me a sister, that living at Grandma's was not a choice I had to make so many years earlier.

Chapter 17

My New Aerodynamic Body

Most of the important things in the world have been accomplished by people who have kept on trying when there seemed to be no hope at all.
Dale Carnegie

On the third day after surgery, I was sent home to start life as a "gutted" female. I thought I knew exactly how I would feel coming home, but it was still a shocker. I became a statistic instead of a person. I was not Anita DuJardin Hockers: wife, mother, sister, daughter, employee, college graduate, etc. I was Hockers, A. Cancer patient.

As great as all the care I received was, it seemed as if the hospital staff went about its business in a very detached way. They opened me up, took out just about every female part I had, and then sent me home as soon as they could. *"You're on your way. Best of luck. You'll be just fine. We have others that need our attention now."*

Please don't misunderstand what I am trying to say. They were truly caring to me. The nurses were always there with a smile, a nice warm blanket, and some good pain medication. But, no matter how much you wanted to be able to reach them, they seemed a bit distant. Now I understand why; they had to. If nurses become attached to every person they encounter and care for, how hard would that be for them?

They need to stay one step away, emotionally, for their own self-preservation.

I said very little on the ride home. When we turned the corner onto Arrowhead Drive, I started to cry. It was a winter wonderland. The snow was piled up along the driveways, and the trees had that surreal frosted look I love. There was a snowman in the neighbor's yard and a few icicles hanging from the porch roof. I took it all in as Ray helped me into the house and upstairs to our bedroom. *I'm home. I'm finally, really and truly home.* Mom was there, ready as always to help me if I needed anything.

I took a nap and then told Ray I wanted to take a shower. After lying in a hospital bed for four days, I needed to be clean. I just had to get clean. It was like the water ritual in Christian churches where they baptize people to wash away their sins. I needed to cleanse myself of all I had endured, to wash what had happened to me down the drain. But I could hardly stand up straight, let alone take a shower.

I tried with all my might to spare Ray this extra work, but I couldn't. I just stood there helpless, crying. I will never forget a single detail of what happened next. It was one of the most wonderful, caring moments of my life.

Ray smiled patiently as he helped me undress and get into the shower. Then he watched me so I wouldn't fall. I wasn't sure if I had the legs to stand. Ray wasn't sure how to hold me, so he stayed close enough to catch me.

"You're still the only girl for me, Anita," he said while I watched the warm water run over my new flat chest. I couldn't actually feel the water because my chest was numb, but it was so relaxing. Ray said, "I love you, Anita, and nothing else matters." Then he added, "You're just more aerodynamic, honey. Now you're built for speed."

Isn't that something? I was stripped of almost everything a female needs to call herself sexy, and Ray still thought I was a hot babe. Who wouldn't love this incredible man?

There was another way that Ray was almost heroic in his efforts to care for me. I was sent home from the hospital with those four drain tubes still connected to my body. The idea is that the suction or vacuum at the end of each of the compacted bulbs pulls the excess fluid out; then it is collected and discarded. If not for these drains, my chest would most likely have filled with fluid.

As Dr. Colette had predicted, my drains continued to collect fluid for about two weeks. This is good; the negative part is that the accumulated fluids have to be emptied or "stripped" twice each day. Ray was not exactly thrilled about the prospect, but he knew I could not do it myself.

Stripping a drain consists of taking something skinny and flat, like a pencil or pen, and holding the spot where the drain exits your skin, and pulling the fluid in the lines down to the collection bulb. The collected matter—blood, clots and other body fluids—wasn't pretty, but the process is amazing. Despite the fact that this task is distasteful at best, Ray did not complain once.

The first day I was home, I asked Mom if she wanted to see my chest. Call it morbid curiosity, but I watch people's faces when they look. Mom showed no shock, just a little wince from a mother who knew her daughter was hurting.

Most people want to see my chest, but do not feel they dare ask. So I ask them if they would like to take a look, and I show everyone who wants to. In fact, Ray says, "Man, are you ever going to keep your shirt on?"

Some people say that I show them my chest because it's therapy for me. I disagree. I show everyone who wants to look because one in seven women will have breast cancer. People NEED to know what can happen. I certainly did not know what it would look like. If I can show others that my chest is really not that bad, maybe that will be one less fear the next victim will have to deal with.

Recovering from surgery has always been pretty easy for me. I have never done much lying around, and I consider myself a fast-healer. This time wasn't much different. It was so much easier than recovering from chemotherapy. I needed my rest, so I napped when I could. But in a few days, I was feeling much better. I was also in pretty good spirits. My family and friends kept me pretty busy so I didn't have much time for self-pity. My friends took me out to lunch, and the boys at work brought me lunch. Believe me, I did not go hungry!

One of my first outings during my recovery was to have my drains removed. Dr. Colette had told me she would just pull them out, quickly, when my chest was done draining. I was terrified. As I said earlier, the drains had been inserted into my body after surgery. They were still there, about six inches below my armpit. I could actually feel part of the drain near my collarbone. How could she just "pull" them out?

There was a fresh layer of snow that day. Mom was an hour away at her home in Egg Harbor, and I didn't want her driving on slippery roads. Colleen was three hours away in Chicago. Ray was very busy trying to seal a deal, and I was afraid to go alone. I needed someone to hold my hand. I called Brenda Brice.

I met Brenda eight years ago while sitting at the YMCA watching our boys swim. Brenda has been a special blessing. She's the type of person who makes you smile and feel good every time you're with her. We connected and began to talk every month or so. Little did we know as we sat on the benches at the YMCA, that our husbands had known each other through their businesses in the construction industry. The four of us have shared many a margarita the past couple of years. Our friendship has always been the kind where you feel totally relaxed.

I'd had lunch with Brenda in June 2004 and had taken her to the new house to show her the size of the project. She was impressed by our ambition and completely understood why we didn't have time to get together or chat during construction. Still, she said she had been thinking of me when I called her that August. When I told her about the diagnosis, she was floored. "It was like a punch to the stomach," she explained to me later. But she ratcheted up her courage, put on a happy face, and came over the next day with a plate of cookies. She has been there for me ever since.

Being a cancer patient sucks, but all we really need is for someone to be there, someone to count on, with no strings attached. Brenda was all that and more. She made time for me; she knew what I needed. Whether it was calling to check on me, making cookies for Ray and the kids, or bringing me books to read, Brenda did it without fail. So when it was time to have the drains removed, I called her. "Brenda, can you come over and take me for a ride?"

She laughed and said, "Anytime, but where are we going?"

"Gotta get these drains out," I said nervously. She was there in an hour.

I took two anti-anxiety pills and two aspirin. It crossed my mind that it was over-kill (and it was), but I had no idea what to expect when we arrived at the clinic. Brenda looked at me and smiled as we were ushered into the examining room. I gave her a weak one back. Dr. Colette's nurse came in and said, "This won't take long at all. You might be more comfortable on the table though, lying down."

I held Brenda's hand tightly and closed my eyes. The nurse counted to three and gently eased the drains out. I felt no pain. I am not kidding. There was a weird sensation, a quick burn, but no pain. I opened my eyes and Brenda was beaming. *No problem at all.*

I did encounter a small complication about a week after all four drains were out. The right side of my chest started to fill up with fluid. This, compared to everything else, made me very sick. I touched my chest and it gurgled, like touching a waterbed without baffles. I knew this was serious and called

Dr. Colette, who saw me that very day. She inserted a large syringe into my incision line and removed a significant amount of fluid from my chest.

I wanted to ask her how much fluid she had removed, but decided against it when I stood up. The massiveness of what I had been through was hitting home. I felt faint and weak; I just wanted to go back to bed. There were no questions: I had just enough energy for a small smile and, "I'll see you soon." After that, my body took care of itself and absorbed the excess fluid on its own. I will always think that my body must have known that I didn't want to have that procedure done again!

The next outing for Brenda and me was to pick out my new boobs. Now this is **not** a shopping trip on which you ask just anyone to accompany you. It's not like calling a friend and saying, "Let's go grab a cup of coffee." Or "Let's go see that new chick flick." Or even, "Will you help me find the perfect mother-of-the-bride dress?" No, this is just plain weird. "Will you take me shopping? I need you to help me pick out my new boobs."

This wasn't my first shopping foray to find my "new look." Mom and I had gone to see what the "next best thing" was when I was undergoing chemotherapy. I was concerned about the weight of prosthetic breasts, determined to find the most realistic, lightest ones around. There was one problem. How could I try on boobs while I still had my own? We gave it a shot anyway. I found some I thought would work. So Mom and I had chosen the type of prosthetic, but just not the size.

You cannot imagine what it's like to come to the realization that you need to buy yourself a prosthetic pair of boobs. I know this may sound hypocritical, but even though I had definitely decided not to reconstruct my breasts, I still wanted to LOOK like a woman. Brenda understood completely, and off we went to pick out my boobs.

When you think of prosthetics, you think of artificial arms and legs, not breasts. It was a bit awkward at first. I was nervous, and as per usual, I made jokes. We giggled a LOT. I tried some on that were too small, which was absolutely hilarious because we were so used to seeing me with a large chest. We tried some on that looked like torpedoes. If it had been the 1950s, I would have fit right in. Brenda smiled with me when we found some that would probably be all right. We ordered them.

"Yes, I would like those in Caucasian, triangle shape, small C." You would have thought I was ordering from a specialty restaurant menu. We giggled again.

When I tell people I am a breast cancer survivor, the first thing they do is look at my chest. It's only a fleeting glance, and it's quite a normal thing to do, but I am always amused by their reaction, or rather, lack of one. Mom, Brenda, and I must have picked out some good ones all right. No one can tell the difference.

Chapter 18
I Don't Want to Hurt Anymore

Dwelling on the negative simply contributes to its power.
Shirley MacLaine

Radiation therapy began on February 17, six months after I had discovered that first lump. My radiation oncologist and Dr. Colette both recommended it. The reason? Remember, during the sentinel node biopsy in August, two of my lymph nodes tested positive, an indication that the cancer was moving out of the breast to invade other parts of my body. Even though the PET scan showed no other hot spots, and the pathology reports showed no cancer cells after the mastectomy, everyone wanted to be sure.

I have to admit that at first I was afraid. Mom had told me that Grandma Evelyn had also undergone radiation treatment in her fight against cancer. Mom didn't know many details; talking about such things wasn't "proper" in the 1950s. But Mom did say that Grandma's burns were extensive and very disfiguring. When Grandpa Pete learned that he had cancer in his eighties, he refused radiation treatment. All he could think of was Grandma Evelyn's horrible experience.

However, as with so many medical treatments today, the procedures are much more sophisticated and do considerably less collateral damage. The technicians have better equipment and much more control than they did 50 years ago. Thus, for more than a month, I dutifully reported for radiation. Once again, I surrendered control to total strangers, people who would burn my flesh with ultra high-energy waves in their pursuit of a higher goal: saving my life. Again, I willingly put my body and my life into the hands of those who are lumped together under the term "health care professionals."

Health care *professionals*. Man…you better believe they were professional. The nurses and technicians in radiation therapy were incredible. They witness horrible sickness and dreadful scars, but they proceed with their work because they know they provide a victim's last line of defense. They understand how emotional it is, and they perform their duties with patience, good humor, and encouragement. I remember one particularly kind nurse named Gloria who said, "This is your last battle, Anita. Get through this and it's over. You're done." *Oh, how I want this to be over and done!*

Before my treatment could begin, my radiation oncologist took measurements of my chest. He analyzed the measurements to get the correct angle for radiation, then checked my charts to determine the proper dose. The nurses permanently tattooed four marks on my chest to use as guides for lining up the high-energy waves. These marks would be the target area. Daily positioning of the machine needs to be accurate, and the tattoos are their guide. Four tattoos, four more battle souvenirs. *All I can say is, why in the hell would people freely choose to get a tattoo? It hurts!*

Once I was "marked," they lined me up every day, Monday through Friday, for 33 days. The object was to kill any cancer cells that might still be lurking in my body. Just the massive size of the machine is intimidating. It's HUGE, with an arm that swings and pivots around you. The nurses asked me to remove my shirt and my "new boobs." I put on a hospital gown and was then instructed to lie down on a flat table.

"Okay Anita, stay as still as you can. We're going to line you up," Gloria said as she and her assistant used laser lines directed at my tattoos to position my body in the exact spot necessary for the radiation to properly do its job.

"Now, we're going to leave the room. But we'll be close by."

"Why are you leaving?" I asked nervously, my eyes darting all over the room. I had no idea what was going to happen and I thought that it might hurt. I didn't want to hurt anymore.

"We have to...the radiation...we can't be exposed." They smiled and left, shutting an enormous door behind them. I was terrified even though they had assured me that there would be no pain.

They called to me from the other room. "Anita, are you all right?"

"Yup, you bet I am." Nervous laughter followed. *Typical me.*

"We're watching you; we promise." They were indeed watching me...through closed-circuit television cameras. The entire treatment took less than three minutes. Just like an ordinary x-ray, there is absolutely no pain involved. It took longer to get undressed than it did to radiate my chest.

Nervous giggles again when they came back in with smiling faces and high praise. "You did just great." The tears came fast. I was so relieved.

Radiation went really well until the last week. After all, this is a radical medical procedure, and there are side effects even if it doesn't hurt. The treatment can cause a wide array of physical symptoms associated with radiation sickness. Some people are excessively tired. Some have nausea. Some get infections. Sometimes the side effect is psychological: depression. My only negative reaction until that last week was minor fatigue. I kept thinking, *This isn't that bad. It's nothing compared to chemotherapy and surgery.*

But you can't burn your body every day for over a month and not have *something* negative happen. By the last week, my burns, which were only on the right side where the tumors were, were pretty sore and leaking. It was painful to stand, to sit, and especially to lie down. I kept thinking how agonizing it must be to suffer severe burns in an accident, during wartime, or as a crime victim.

I also thought often of Grandma Evelyn, remembering the stories I had heard about this brave, beautiful woman. How I would have loved to talk to her, to compare notes on what was happening to me. As I thought of her fight with cancer, I kept coming to the same conclusion. Although I was hurting something awful, my pain was nothing compared to hers.

I did my best to minimize the chance of anything going wrong on my account. I was scrupulous about hygiene; I did not want to get an infection. Therefore, I did everything the nurses told me to do: wash my hands well; cleanse the area thoroughly; apply topical burn ointments. My diligence paid off. Eventually my burns healed very nicely. The skin that covers the treated area is a bit darker than the rest of my chest, but hey, that's really minor.

Seven and a half months after diagnosis, it was finally over. I had reached the finish line. I completed the last battle of my personal war against cancer. Seven and a half months of my life; it's hard to get my arms around that.

I can't end this chapter without telling you about a young woman I met during this time period. Her name is Paula VandenHeuvel. She had neck and throat cancer and was undergoing radiation after her surgery. She was so scared and so terribly sick. Because of the radiation treatments to her neck, her salivary glands had shut down. She needed to be hospitalized because she could not swallow. Her only means of nutrition was through an IV bag on a pole. Intravenous feedings were her lifeline.

I so wanted to convince her that everything was going to be all right. I needed to give her strength, the same strength that Lorene had given me. On one of Paula's particularly bad days, I told her, "Don't let anyone tell you that this cancer stuff doesn't suck rocks, because it does. But we are going to make it through this, Paula. I know we will." She has told me on more than one occasion how much my words meant to her. She had been tempted to give up; she was so tired, but the sheer force of my will to live was contagious.

Yes, even though some days I wanted to sit and cry or stand and scream, I would walk down the hall to radiation treatment, bald head held high, sunglasses on, with a determined smile on my face. Paula says my positive attitude helped her. It put the sunshine of a smile into her dreary day. And believe me, it helped me, too.

Paula and her mom surprised me on my last day of radiation with a dozen pink roses. Paula had finished her radiation therapy two weeks earlier. She was bravely trying to get back to normal, but she was still so very weak from lack of nutrition. Somehow, she managed to get showered, buy flowers, and meet me at the hospital. I was overwhelmed. Paula and her mother did not even know me, but they were concerned and really cared about the success of my recovery.

Paula's mom confided that my "sucks rocks" comment was inspirational to their whole family. (Imagine that kind of language being inspirational!) "There was so much sadness in Paula before you talked to her," she said. "She needed to hear from another cancer survivor that it was all right to feel bad. It was okay to be angry, sad, even resentful, but to never, ever give up."

My mom and Paula's mother hugged for a long time that afternoon. During that long month, our mothers had bonded as only women can when they have a lot of painful experiences in common. They did not talk much, but knew with just a glance that their sadness for their daughters was a shared emotion. Their children were sick, and they were helpless. All they could do was love us.

Chapter 19
We're More Than the Sum of Our Parts

Nothing can bring you peace but yourself.
Ralph Waldo Emerson

You learn a lot during those long months of suffering, lying there in bed with only the pain and your thoughts to reassure you that you are still alive. You learn that nothing is more important than making time in your life for the people that matter. You learn that, although you are entitled to wallow in self-pity, it makes no sense to feel sorry for yourself because it doesn't do one single solitary thing to make your treatment and recovery easier.

Not that "strong" Anita is completely immune to an occasional attack of self-pity. Toward the end of my treatment, my body and mind were so weakened that it was hard to resist. I started thinking too much and began feeling resentful. I was so sure that the world should have stopped when I was diagnosed. I wanted it to be like a merry-go-round. Stop, let me get my business with this cancer-thing done, and then start the world back up again. How dare people go on with their lives when mine was unraveling at the seams? I suppose I was entitled to those thoughts, but now I think it was more that I wanted and needed to get back to living.

And so I did. I still live in our dream house on beautiful tree-lined Arrowhead Drive in Green Bay. My daughter is in high school, and my son in middle school. Ray still thinks I'm the only girl for him, and he will get no argument from me on that score. Our family is still close, and Colleen and I talk, email, and see each other as often as possible. I still make time for my friends, play volleyball, go to Packer games, and scream my lungs out whether they win or lose. I still work at FedEx Ground, and I still enjoy a cocktail with my chips and salsa at Los Banditos.

Thank goodness I had health insurance to cover my illness and did not have THAT worry, too. Treating breast cancer is expensive. I was sick over two years, which meant that I had two deductibles to meet and two out-of-pocket-cost thresholds to reach, but there are NO complaints from me. What's a life worth?

Ribbon of Hope, an organization for breast cancer victims, helped me emotionally and financially. Lorene had told me that they had helped her, but I was a bit reluctant to ask. Ray and I could have found one way or another to clean up our medical bills, but Kathy, Meg and Linda—the Ribbon of Hope founders—were insistent. They explained that the organization is there to help all breast cancer victims, no matter their situation. Each breast cancer patient is allotted a set dollar amount to help pay for any service incurred while undergoing treatment. Their support was a ray of sunshine, and I hope that one day I can give them as much as they gave me.

In the process of recording my recent life challenges, I have come to some very intriguing realizations. I never thought I would say this, but I recommend that anyone going through a really rough time in life should write about it. Writing this book made me aware that we as humans have to let go of things in order to move on. The wondrous part is that what we let go of often comes back in a new and better way.

Let me explain. Going to college and letting go of my safety net made me realize how much I enjoy being home. It made me responsible, in charge of my own life, but it also reinforced my need to be with family. When I was in high school, cheering, making friends, growing up, I let go of some of the sister connection I had with Colleen. But my cancer solidified and strengthened our relationship in a way I could not have imagined possible. Going through this illness forced me to let go and stop controlling things. I had to let the powers that be lead me on my path. Abandoning my need to control everything when I was sick was a must. That brought incredible rewards: new friends, new experiences, and a wonderful appreciation of what really matters. Having perfect breasts is one of the things that doesn't.

This world is unbelievably hooked on the perfect female body. We are constantly bombarded by the images of beautiful women. They dazzle us with their perfect teeth, their perfect skin, their perfect legs, their tiny waistlines, their perky, surgically enhanced breasts. Whether it's movies, television, magazines, posters, billboards, or advertising brochures, these airbrushed, unnatural beauties smile at us, seemingly content in their perfect bodies.

Of course, there are times, now that my surgery is more than a year behind me, that I still get angry. And sad. It was a life-altering experience. Then again, even if I had boobs, I would never look like those women. Even if I had never had breast cancer, I would have never looked like them. Perfect breasts, pencil-thin legs, flat stomach…this has never been me. What's more, my disease is testament to the fact that physical beauty is merely a fleeting illusion. It holds no spell over those of us who have gone into the inferno and escaped with our hearts, our minds, and our spirits intact.

Chapter 20

Smile: You're on This Side of the Sod

I have no control over what happens. What I do have control over is how I am going to accept it and move past the challenges.
Anita DuJardin Hockers

Believe it or don't: not having breasts is really no big deal to me. I do not miss them. I am more than my boobs. I always have been. Putting your boobs in the drawer at bedtime is really not all that bad, considering the alternative. As my old friend Marlys used to say, "Hey, we're on this side of the sod, aren't we?"

I do not know, nor do any of us, how much time I have left. I do know I have no time for the negative. It may be a tired old cliché, but it's absolutely true. Life is too short.

When I look back, I realize I haven't changed that much. I am still "crazy Anita." I am still in control and still have to be in charge. I am still loud. I still love my family with all my heart and soul. I still love my Ray and know why I fell for him so long ago. I know who loves me to pieces and vice versa. Only now, I know what's *really* important. The people who are beside me are the things that really matter.

And so my story ends, but, thanks to modern medicine, my family, my friends, my faith, and my life go on. Dr. Colette tells me that if the cancer is to recur, it will probably do so within three years of diagnosis. Three years. I have logged twenty-one months already. I am over half-way there. The prognosis is good.

Why did I have to go through this? I don't know. Maybe it was the right day, maybe the moon was rising, and the stars were aligned at just the right angle. *It was on my path.* I had no control over what happened. What I do have control over is how I am going to accept it and move past the challenges.

And so my choice is to move forward with my head held high, with a positive attitude. I don't show people my chest and my prosthetics for myself; I do it so people will know it's not really that bad. I didn't write this book for myself either. I wrote it for people who are fighting this cancer beast. I wrote it for their loved ones. I wrote it for you, to tell you that you CAN do it, that you will endure, that you will survive. In the final analysis, I may be breastless, but I'm still breathing. That's what counts.

About the Author

Anita Marie DuJardin Hockers was born and raised in Green Bay, Wisconsin. She graduated from the University of Wisconsin–Green Bay with a degree in Marketing and Communications. Anita is a twenty-one month survivor of breast cancer and tries to make every day count with a positive attitude and a smile. She lives in Green Bay with her husband Ray and their two children.

Anita would love to receive your comments about *Breastless But Still Breathing*. You may contact her on-line at breastless@new.rr.com.

Ribbon of Hope
816 Flambeau Place
De Pere, WI 54115
920-337-9192

Ribbon of Hope is a financial, informational, and emotional resource for individuals with breast cancer in Northeastern Wisconsin. Ribbon of Hope helps pay for medical bills, medication, rent, utilities, etc., while a person is receiving treatment for breast cancer. To be eligible for financial assistance, breast cancer patients must live, work, or receive treatment in Brown or Kewaunee counties. Ribbon of Hope financially assists breast cancer patients regardless of age, race, or religion.

Ribbon of Hope Foundation is an all-volunteer organization, and all funds go back into the community to help breast cancer patients. The board consists of breast cancer survivors and spouses dedicated to helping others with this disease. The Board of Directors are Meg M. Fay, Terry Lischka, Kathy & Rick Miller and Linda Rueckl.

www.ribbonofhope.com

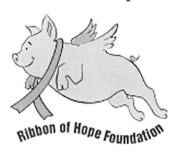

Other books published by Otter Run Books:

My Mother Kept a Scrapbook: the True Story of a WWII POW **(2005)** by Gerhard Johnson. A chilling memoir of a "dogface" army private, this must-read book traces Johnson's horrendous experiences during his imprisonment in German Prison Stalag IIB. It is supported by newspaper clippings, letters, telegrams, and war bulletins his mother gathered in a valiant effort to keep her son "alive" as long as she could.

Sunrise Sunset **(2004)** by Heather Sprangers and Kathleen Marie Marsh is an inspirational mainstream novel that traces the circle of life from infertility to Alzheimer's Disease. This poignant novel, which depicts a heart-warming story of cross-generational friendship, is a tribute to the many ways women have of weathering life's storms.

The Portly Princess of Thynneland **(2004)** by Kathleen Marie Marsh is an enchanting fairy tale for grown-ups that addresses the critical role parents play in preventing childhood obesity. This hardcover, illustrated, delightful little book depicts the adventures, romance and heroic exploits of Volumina, an overweight princess living in a country where being fat is illegal.

The Portly Princess of Thinland **(2006)** by Kathleen Marie Marsh is a hilariously entertaining romp with a timely message. A musical comedy stage play perfect for high school or community college venues, this play gently reminds parents of their responsibility in developing healthy eating habits in their children. (Script, music and costumes available).